THE
BEAUTY
EDITOR'S
WORKBOOK

THE BEAUTY EDITOR'S WORKBOOK

Felicia Milewicz and Lois Joy Johnson

Illustrated by Lois Joy Johnson

Random House New York

Personal acknowledgments

We wish to offer special thanks to the following people for everything they have taught us over the years: Rex Hilverdink, make-up artist; Lydia Sarfati, owner and president of Klisar Skin Care; hair experts Pascal Boissier, Gerard Bollei, Howard Fugler, Didier Malige and John Sahag. We also wish to acknowledge with gratitude the assistance given to us by our editor, Klara Glowczewski.

To my mother, to my best friend and dear husband, Marek, and my son Jasio.

—Felicia

To my daughter, Jennifer Jolie.

—Lois

Library of Congress Cataloging in Publication Data

Milewicz, Felicia.
The beauty editor's workbook.

Includes index.
1. Beauty, Personal.   I. Johnson, Lois.
II. Title.
RA778.M57 1983   646.7'042   82-42825
ISBN 0-394-71533-0

Manufactured in the United States of America

98765432

First Edition

Foreword

Beauty . . . that elusive quality pursued by women of all ages, throughout the ages. It's a world unto itself . . . and it welcomes you to relax, open your mind, and explore its not-so-mysterious secrets.

Today, more than ever before, beauty is a mirror reflection of your lifestyle and attitudes. A sensible, healthy foundation of exercise, nutrition, and rest is vital to the success of even the most sensational hairstyle or make-up. The way you look announces loud and clear how you feel; the magic word is "confidence."

Why? Because beauty is basic and that's exactly how our book deals with it. Our purpose is to help you develop a strong sense of beauty confidence by showing you exactly *what* to do, as well as *when* and *how* to do it. Our approach is straightforward and simple—with an emphasis on *fun*—so that your approach to beauty can be the same.

Until recently, beauty experts directed their advice to "types"; to achieve a particular look, you wore a particular shade of lipstick, blush, and eye shadow, and you styled your hair in a particular way. Today's woman, whatever her age, knows she doesn't have to settle for a "type." She's an individual with needs and tastes of her own. Her beauty regimen should not be dictated by what the Hollywood star of the moment or her best friend is wearing, but should be viewed as an exploration of herself . . . taking into consideration all the special components that make her who she is.

This book will help you discover and fully develop your own personal beauty sense. Who knows? The nose that seems a little too long or the brows that seem a little too full might turn out to be one of your most interesting assets. You don't have to be an artist to look beautiful. With simple basics, we'll teach you to be comfortable with the world of beauty and learn to use it as a means of self-expression.

But, even more importantly, you'll have fun. Beauty shouldn't be viewed as a serious learning process, and that's why this book doesn't make you plod through pages and pages of words. We know that your time is at a premium. When you want information you want it fast, and we've put everything right at your fingertips with clear, simple illustrations.

The Beauty Editor's Workbook is a visual encyclopedia of beauty, with each chapter devoted to a specific aspect: facial care, make-up, hair care, hair styling, and body care. Just flip to the right section and you'll quickly find the answers you're looking for. It's a "beauty game" that's meant to be thoroughly enjoyed. And the beauty of it is that *you* always come out a winner!

So, welcome to the world of beauty. It is our pleasure to share with you these personal notes and observations acquired over our many years of experience in the beauty field. We dedicate this book to you—those exploring beauty for the first time and those rediscovering it—and invite you to become your most beautiful you.

Felicia Milewicz   *Lois Joy Johnson*

How to Use This Book

The Beauty Editor's Workbook is divided into five chapters: 1) Facial Care, 2) Make-up, 3) Hair Care, 4) Hair Styling, 5) Body Care. The drawings and captions within each chapter are numbered sequentially, each chapter beginning with #1. You can go through an entire chapter by simply following the numbers: just look at the drawings, read the captions, and experiment with the beauty methods and ideas we suggest. Or, if you want a quick answer to a specific question or problem, simply flip to the directory of subjects at the beginning of each chapter: you will find a list of the specific topics covered in the chapter, and the drawing and caption numbers that pertain to them (in each chapter the number of the drawing and caption that begins a new topic is backed by a red circle, for easy reference). Or, you can browse through the entire book, flipping to this page or that, looking, reading, trying the various techniques, discovering new ways to make yourself look fabulous. We urge you to use the *Workbook* in all three ways.

CONTENTS

Introduction:

CONSIDER YOUR FACE

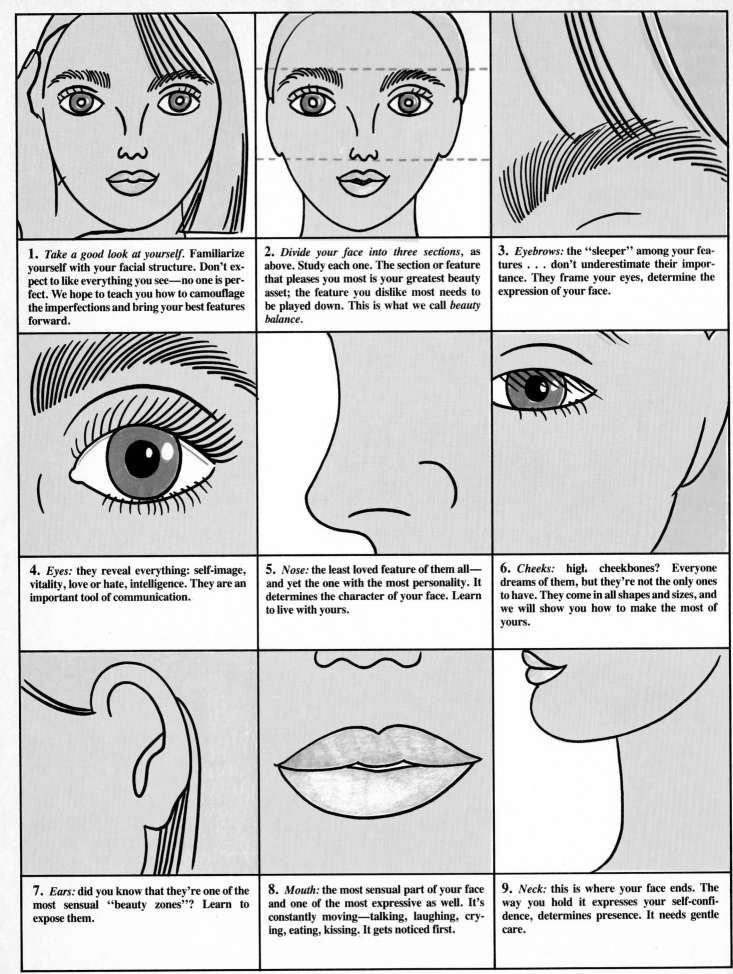

1. *Take a good look at yourself.* Familiarize yourself with your facial structure. Don't expect to like everything you see—no one is perfect. We hope to teach you how to camouflage the imperfections and bring your best features forward.

2. *Divide your face into three sections,* as above. Study each one. The section or feature that pleases you most is your greatest beauty asset; the feature you dislike most needs to be played down. This is what we call *beauty balance.*

3. *Eyebrows:* the "sleeper" among your features . . . don't underestimate their importance. They frame your eyes, determine the expression of your face.

4. *Eyes:* they reveal everything: self-image, vitality, love or hate, intelligence. They are an important tool of communication.

5. *Nose:* the least loved feature of them all—and yet the one with the most personality. It determines the character of your face. Learn to live with yours.

6. *Cheeks:* high cheekbones? Everyone dreams of them, but they're not the only ones to have. They come in all shapes and sizes, and we will show you how to make the most of yours.

7. *Ears:* did you know that they're one of the most sensual "beauty zones"? Learn to expose them.

8. *Mouth:* the most sensual part of your face and one of the most expressive as well. It's constantly moving—talking, laughing, crying, eating, kissing. It gets noticed first.

9. *Neck:* this is where your face ends. The way you hold it expresses your self-confidence, determines presence. It needs gentle care.

1
FACIAL
CARE

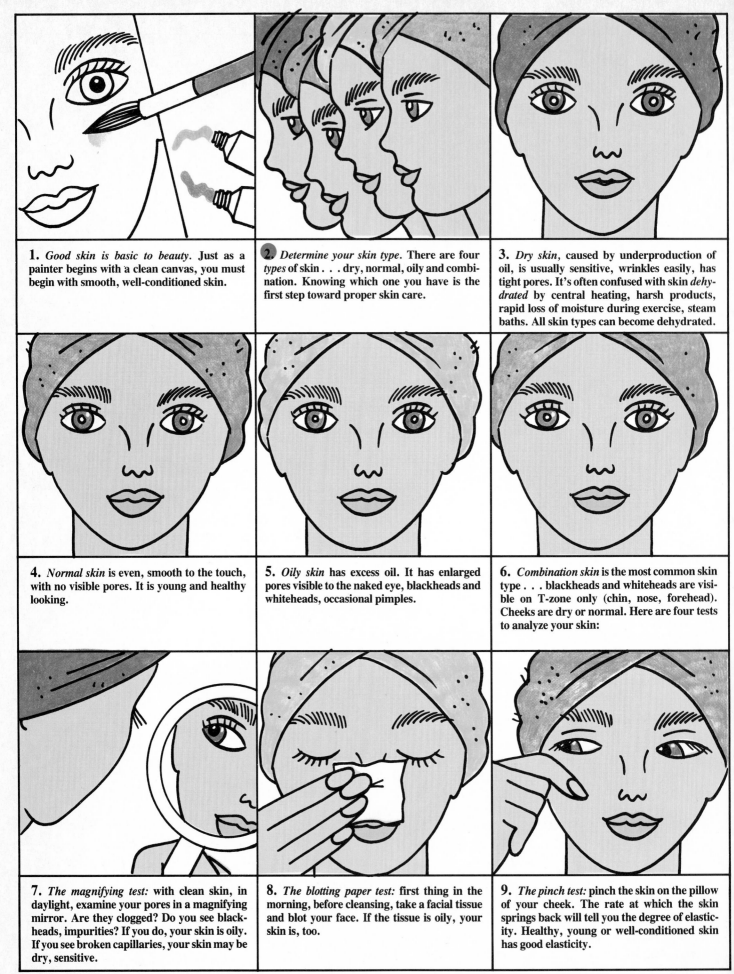

1. *Good skin is basic to beauty.* Just as a painter begins with a clean canvas, you must begin with smooth, well-conditioned skin.

2. *Determine your skin type.* There are four *types* of skin . . . dry, normal, oily and combination. Knowing which one you have is the first step toward proper skin care.

3. *Dry skin*, caused by underproduction of oil, is usually sensitive, wrinkles easily, has tight pores. It's often confused with skin *dehydrated* by central heating, harsh products, rapid loss of moisture during exercise, steam baths. All skin types can become dehydrated.

4. *Normal skin* is even, smooth to the touch, with no visible pores. It is young and healthy looking.

5. *Oily skin* has excess oil. It has enlarged pores visible to the naked eye, blackheads and whiteheads, occasional pimples.

6. *Combination skin* is the most common skin type . . . blackheads and whiteheads are visible on T-zone only (chin, nose, forehead). Cheeks are dry or normal. Here are four tests to analyze your skin:

7. *The magnifying test:* with clean skin, in daylight, examine your pores in a magnifying mirror. Are they clogged? Do you see blackheads, impurities? If you do, your skin is oily. If you see broken capillaries, your skin may be dry, sensitive.

8. *The blotting paper test:* first thing in the morning, before cleansing, take a facial tissue and blot your face. If the tissue is oily, your skin is, too.

9. *The pinch test:* pinch the skin on the pillow of your cheek. The rate at which the skin springs back will tell you the degree of elasticity. Healthy, young or well-conditioned skin has good elasticity.

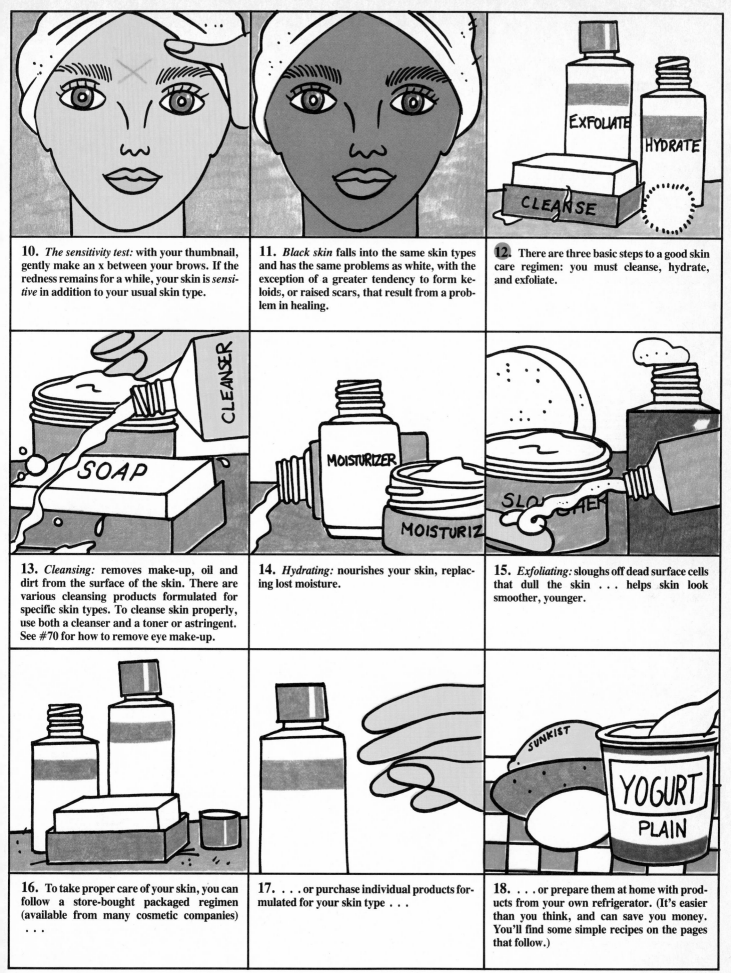

10. *The sensitivity test:* with your thumbnail, gently make an x between your brows. If the redness remains for a while, your skin is *sensitive* in addition to your usual skin type.

11. *Black skin* falls into the same skin types and has the same problems as white, with the exception of a greater tendency to form keloids, or raised scars, that result from a problem in healing.

12. There are three basic steps to a good skin care regimen: you must cleanse, hydrate, and exfoliate.

13. *Cleansing:* removes make-up, oil and dirt from the surface of the skin. There are various cleansing products formulated for specific skin types. To cleanse skin properly, use both a cleanser and a toner or astringent. See #70 for how to remove eye make-up.

14. *Hydrating:* nourishes your skin, replacing lost moisture.

15. *Exfoliating:* sloughs off dead surface cells that dull the skin . . . helps skin look smoother, younger.

16. To take proper care of your skin, you can follow a store-bought packaged regimen (available from many cosmetic companies) . . .

17. . . . or purchase individual products formulated for your skin type . . .

18. . . . or prepare them at home with products from your own refrigerator. (It's easier than you think, and can save you money. You'll find some simple recipes on the pages that follow.)

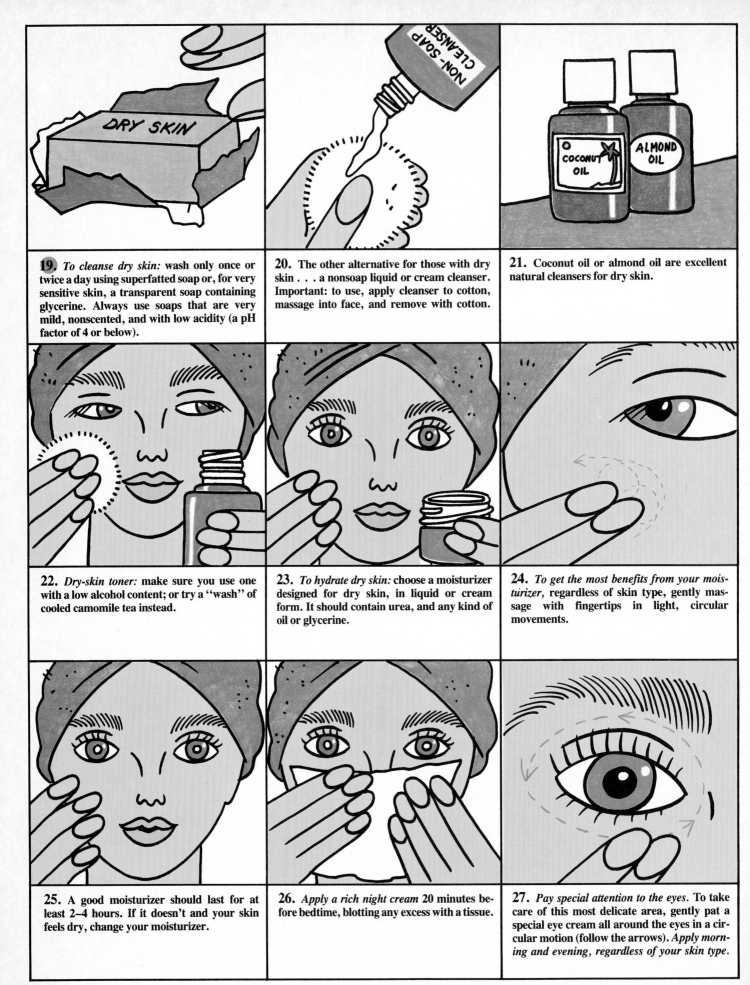

19. *To cleanse dry skin:* wash only once or twice a day using superfatted soap or, for very sensitive skin, a transparent soap containing glycerine. Always use soaps that are very mild, nonscented, and with low acidity (a pH factor of 4 or below).

20. The other alternative for those with dry skin . . . a nonsoap liquid or cream cleanser. Important: to use, apply cleanser to cotton, massage into face, and remove with cotton.

21. Coconut oil or almond oil are excellent natural cleansers for dry skin.

22. *Dry-skin toner:* make sure you use one with a low alcohol content; or try a "wash" of cooled camomile tea instead.

23. *To hydrate dry skin:* choose a moisturizer designed for dry skin, in liquid or cream form. It should contain urea, and any kind of oil or glycerine.

24. *To get the most benefits from your moisturizer,* regardless of skin type, gently massage with fingertips in light, circular movements.

25. A good moisturizer should last for at least 2–4 hours. If it doesn't and your skin feels dry, change your moisturizer.

26. *Apply a rich night cream 20 minutes before bedtime,* blotting any excess with a tissue.

27. *Pay special attention to the eyes.* To take care of this most delicate area, gently pat a special eye cream all around the eyes in a circular motion (follow the arrows). *Apply morning and evening, regardless of your skin type.*

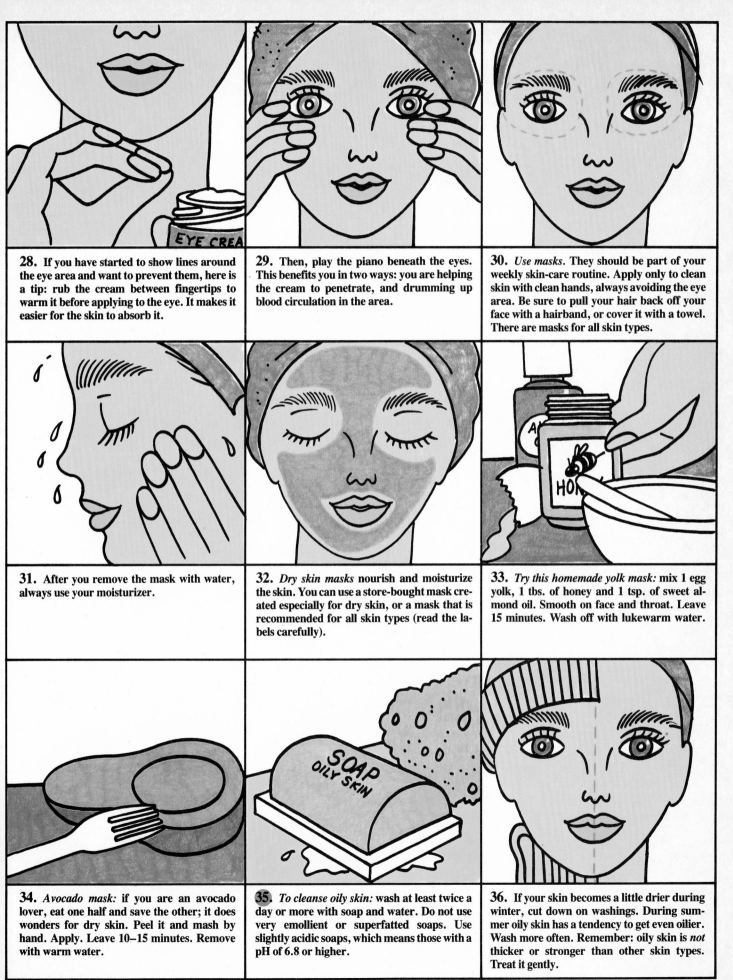

28. If you have started to show lines around the eye area and want to prevent them, here is a tip: rub the cream between fingertips to warm it before applying to the eye. It makes it easier for the skin to absorb it.

29. Then, play the piano beneath the eyes. This benefits you in two ways: you are helping the cream to penetrate, and drumming up blood circulation in the area.

30. *Use masks.* They should be part of your weekly skin-care routine. Apply only to clean skin with clean hands, always avoiding the eye area. Be sure to pull your hair back off your face with a hairband, or cover it with a towel. There are masks for all skin types.

31. After you remove the mask with water, always use your moisturizer.

32. *Dry skin masks* nourish and moisturize the skin. You can use a store-bought mask created especially for dry skin, or a mask that is recommended for all skin types (read the labels carefully).

33. *Try this homemade yolk mask:* mix 1 egg yolk, 1 tbs. of honey and 1 tsp. of sweet almond oil. Smooth on face and throat. Leave 15 minutes. Wash off with lukewarm water.

34. *Avocado mask:* if you are an avocado lover, eat one half and save the other; it does wonders for dry skin. Peel it and mash by hand. Apply. Leave 10–15 minutes. Remove with warm water.

35. *To cleanse oily skin:* wash at least twice a day or more with soap and water. Do not use very emollient or superfatted soaps. Use slightly acidic soaps, which means those with a pH of 6.8 or higher.

36. If your skin becomes a little drier during winter, cut down on washings. During summer oily skin has a tendency to get even oilier. Wash more often. Remember: oily skin is *not* thicker or stronger than other skin types. Treat it gently.

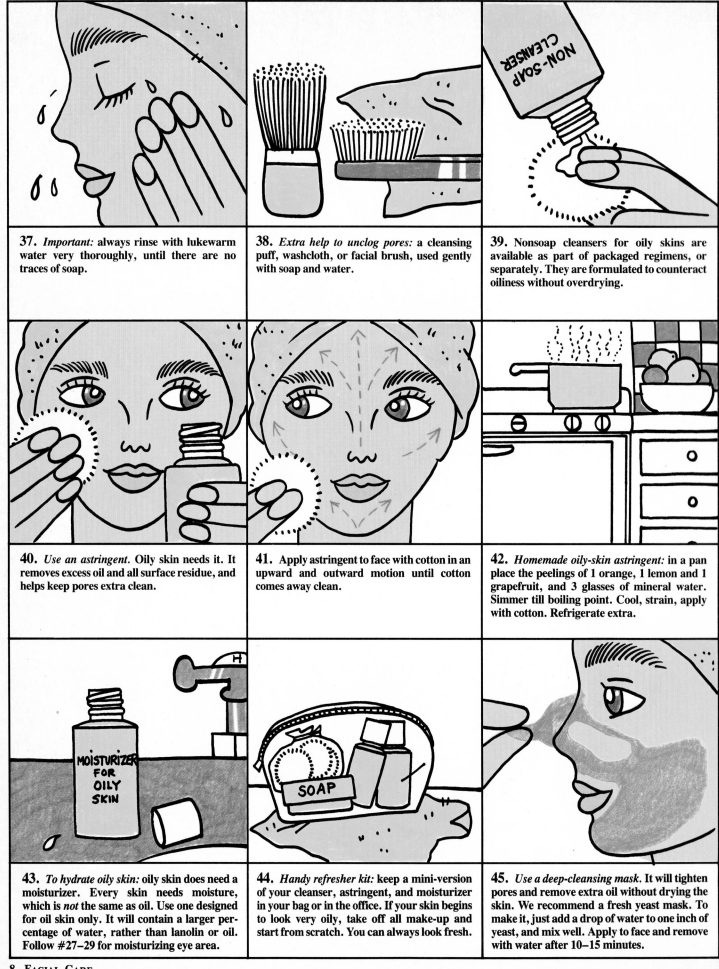

37. *Important:* always rinse with lukewarm water very thoroughly, until there are no traces of soap.

38. *Extra help to unclog pores:* a cleansing puff, washcloth, or facial brush, used gently with soap and water.

39. Nonsoap cleansers for oily skins are available as part of packaged regimens, or separately. They are formulated to counteract oiliness without overdrying.

40. *Use an astringent.* Oily skin needs it. It removes excess oil and all surface residue, and helps keep pores extra clean.

41. Apply astringent to face with cotton in an upward and outward motion until cotton comes away clean.

42. *Homemade oily-skin astringent:* in a pan place the peelings of 1 orange, 1 lemon and 1 grapefruit, and 3 glasses of mineral water. Simmer till boiling point. Cool, strain, apply with cotton. Refrigerate extra.

43. *To hydrate oily skin:* oily skin does need a moisturizer. Every skin needs moisture, which is *not* the same as oil. Use one designed for oil skin only. It will contain a larger percentage of water, rather than lanolin or oil. Follow #27–29 for moisturizing eye area.

44. *Handy refresher kit:* keep a mini-version of your cleanser, astringent, and moisturizer in your bag or in the office. If your skin begins to look very oily, take off all make-up and start from scratch. You can always look fresh.

45. *Use a deep-cleansing mask.* It will tighten pores and remove extra oil without drying the skin. We recommend a fresh yeast mask. To make it, just add a drop of water to one inch of yeast, and mix well. Apply to face and remove with water after 10–15 minutes.

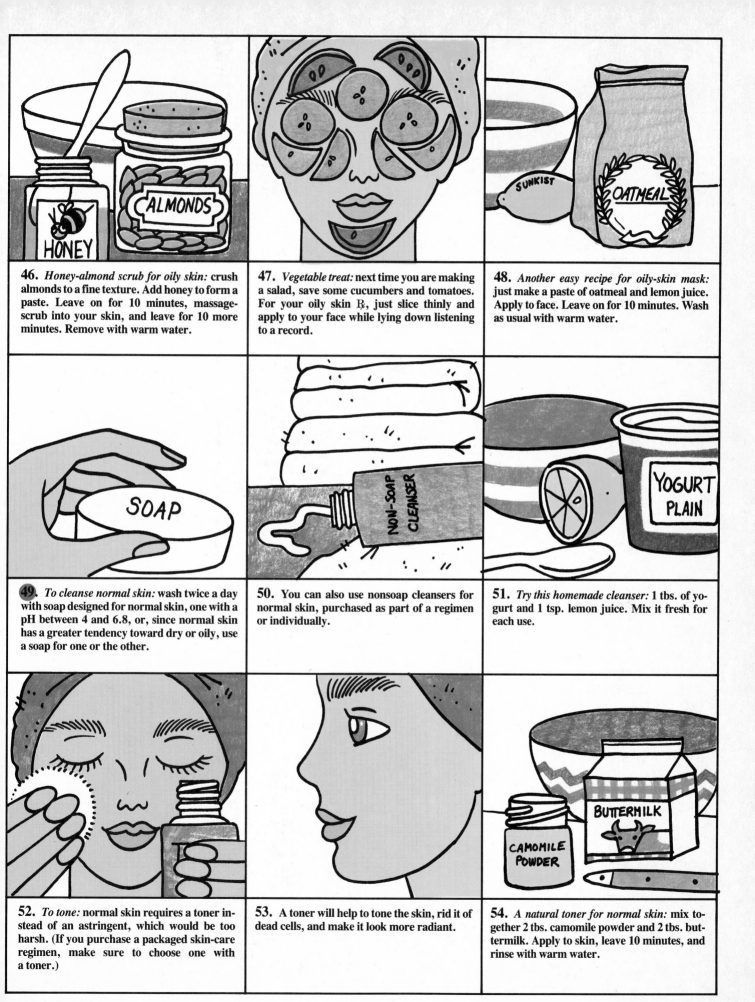

46. *Honey-almond scrub for oily skin:* crush almonds to a fine texture. Add honey to form a paste. Leave on for 10 minutes, massage-scrub into your skin, and leave for 10 more minutes. Remove with warm water.

47. *Vegetable treat:* next time you are making a salad, save some cucumbers and tomatoes. For your oily skin ℞, just slice thinly and apply to your face while lying down listening to a record.

48. *Another easy recipe for oily-skin mask:* just make a paste of oatmeal and lemon juice. Apply to face. Leave on for 10 minutes. Wash as usual with warm water.

49. *To cleanse normal skin:* wash twice a day with soap designed for normal skin, one with a pH between 4 and 6.8, or, since normal skin has a greater tendency toward dry or oily, use a soap for one or the other.

50. You can also use nonsoap cleansers for normal skin, purchased as part of a regimen or individually.

51. *Try this homemade cleanser:* 1 tbs. of yogurt and 1 tsp. lemon juice. Mix it fresh for each use.

52. *To tone:* normal skin requires a toner instead of an astringent, which would be too harsh. (If you purchase a packaged skin-care regimen, make sure to choose one with a toner.)

53. A toner will help to tone the skin, rid it of dead cells, and make it look more radiant.

54. *A natural toner for normal skin:* mix together 2 tbs. camomile powder and 2 tbs. buttermilk. Apply to skin, leave 10 minutes, and rinse with warm water.

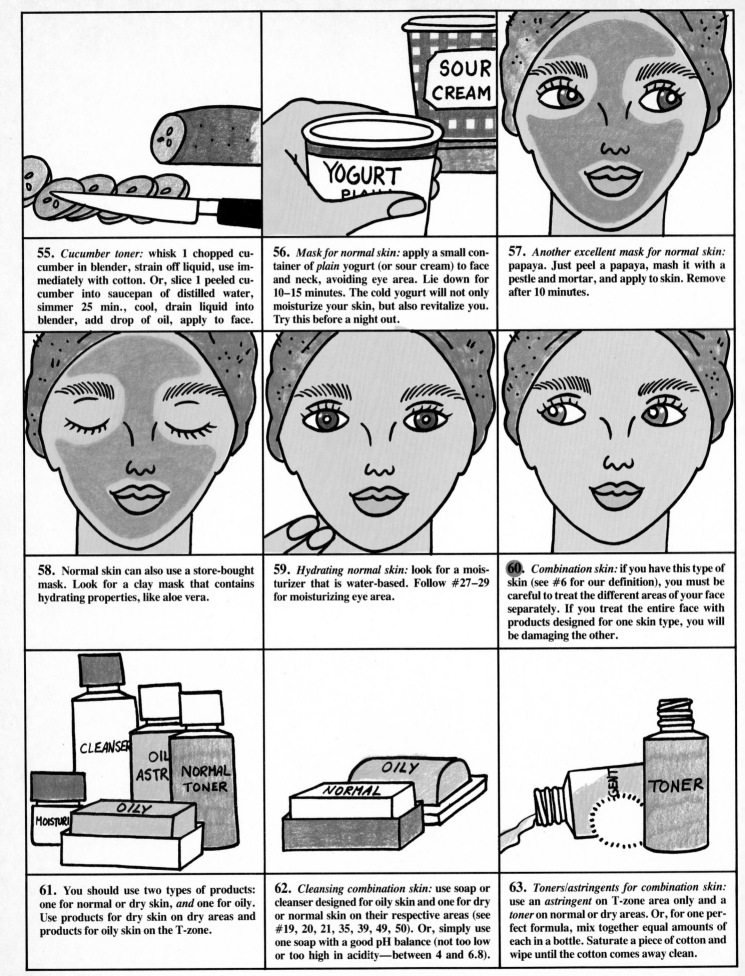

55. *Cucumber toner:* whisk 1 chopped cucumber in blender, strain off liquid, use immediately with cotton. Or, slice 1 peeled cucumber into saucepan of distilled water, simmer 25 min., cool, drain liquid into blender, add drop of oil, apply to face.

56. *Mask for normal skin:* apply a small container of *plain* yogurt (or sour cream) to face and neck, avoiding eye area. Lie down for 10–15 minutes. The cold yogurt will not only moisturize your skin, but also revitalize you. Try this before a night out.

57. *Another excellent mask for normal skin:* papaya. Just peel a papaya, mash it with a pestle and mortar, and apply to skin. Remove after 10 minutes.

58. Normal skin can also use a store-bought mask. Look for a clay mask that contains hydrating properties, like aloe vera.

59. *Hydrating normal skin:* look for a moisturizer that is water-based. Follow #27–29 for moisturizing eye area.

60. *Combination skin:* if you have this type of skin (see #6 for our definition), you must be careful to treat the different areas of your face separately. If you treat the entire face with products designed for one skin type, you will be damaging the other.

61. You should use two types of products: one for normal or dry skin, *and* one for oily. Use products for dry skin on dry areas and products for oily skin on the T-zone.

62. *Cleansing combination skin:* use soap or cleanser designed for oily skin and one for dry or normal skin on their respective areas (see #19, 20, 21, 35, 39, 49, 50). Or, simply use one soap with a good pH balance (not too low or too high in acidity—between 4 and 6.8).

63. *Toners/astringents for combination skin:* use an *astringent* on T-zone area only and a *toner* on normal or dry areas. Or, for one perfect formula, mix together equal amounts of each in a bottle. Saturate a piece of cotton and wipe until the cotton comes away clean.

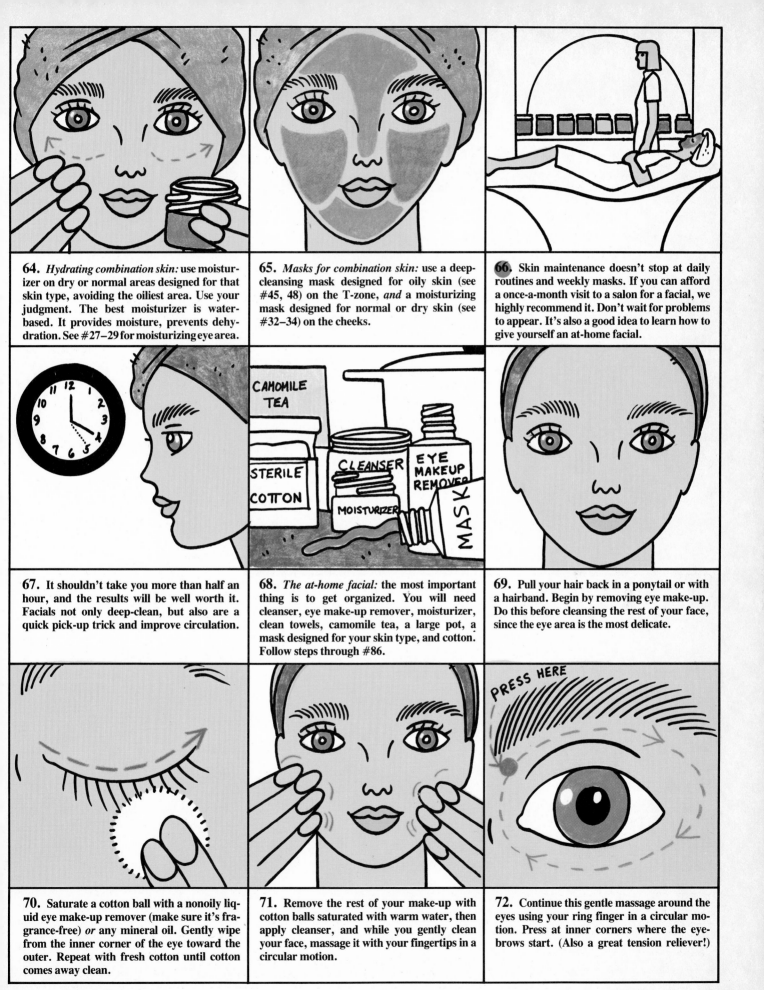

64. *Hydrating combination skin:* use moisturizer on dry or normal areas designed for that skin type, avoiding the oiliest area. Use your judgment. The best moisturizer is water-based. It provides moisture, prevents dehydration. See #27–29 for moisturizing eye area.

65. *Masks for combination skin:* use a deep-cleansing mask designed for oily skin (see #45, 48) on the T-zone, *and* a moisturizing mask designed for normal or dry skin (see #32–34) on the cheeks.

66. Skin maintenance doesn't stop at daily routines and weekly masks. If you can afford a once-a-month visit to a salon for a facial, we highly recommend it. Don't wait for problems to appear. It's also a good idea to learn how to give yourself an at-home facial.

67. It shouldn't take you more than half an hour, and the results will be well worth it. Facials not only deep-clean, but also are a quick pick-up trick and improve circulation.

68. *The at-home facial:* the most important thing is to get organized. You will need cleanser, eye make-up remover, moisturizer, clean towels, camomile tea, a large pot, a mask designed for your skin type, and cotton. Follow steps through #86.

69. Pull your hair back in a ponytail or with a hairband. Begin by removing eye make-up. Do this before cleansing the rest of your face, since the eye area is the most delicate.

70. Saturate a cotton ball with a nonoily liquid eye make-up remover (make sure it's fragrance-free) *or* any mineral oil. Gently wipe from the inner corner of the eye toward the outer. Repeat with fresh cotton until cotton comes away clean.

71. Remove the rest of your make-up with cotton balls saturated with warm water, then apply cleanser, and while you gently clean your face, massage it with your fingertips in a circular motion.

72. Continue this gentle massage around the eyes using your ring finger in a circular motion. Press at inner corners where the eyebrows start. (Also a great tension reliever!)

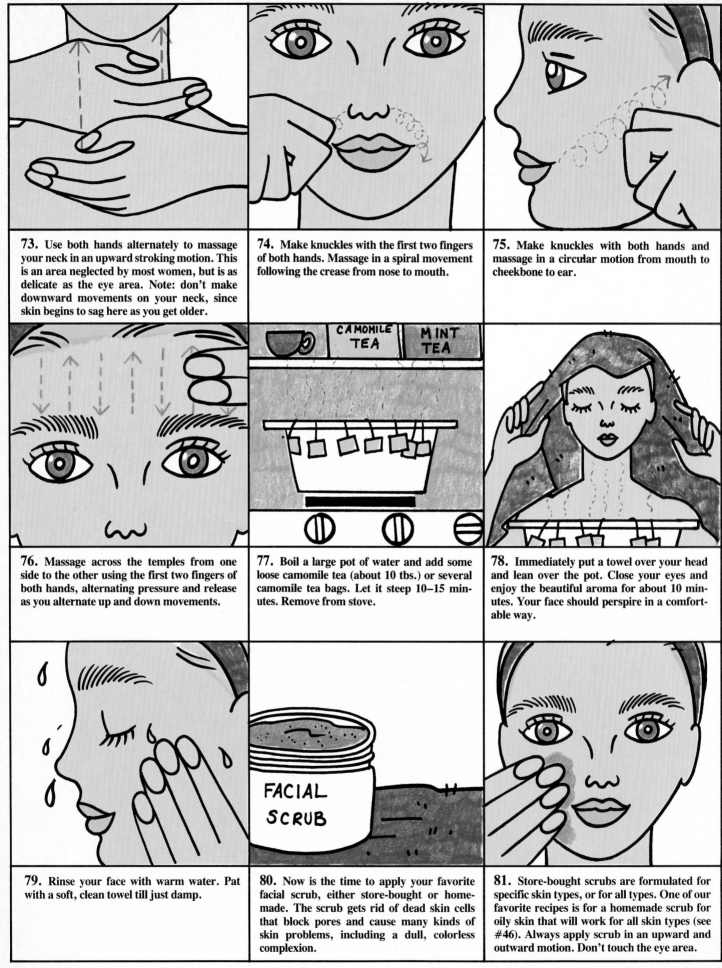

73. Use both hands alternately to massage your neck in an upward stroking motion. This is an area neglected by most women, but is as delicate as the eye area. Note: don't make downward movements on your neck, since skin begins to sag here as you get older.

74. Make knuckles with the first two fingers of both hands. Massage in a spiral movement following the crease from nose to mouth.

75. Make knuckles with both hands and massage in a circular motion from mouth to cheekbone to ear.

76. Massage across the temples from one side to the other using the first two fingers of both hands, alternating pressure and release as you alternate up and down movements.

77. Boil a large pot of water and add some loose camomile tea (about 10 tbs.) or several camomile tea bags. Let it steep 10–15 minutes. Remove from stove.

78. Immediately put a towel over your head and lean over the pot. Close your eyes and enjoy the beautiful aroma for about 10 minutes. Your face should perspire in a comfortable way.

79. Rinse your face with warm water. Pat with a soft, clean towel till just damp.

80. Now is the time to apply your favorite facial scrub, either store-bought or homemade. The scrub gets rid of dead skin cells that block pores and cause many kinds of skin problems, including a dull, colorless complexion.

81. Store-bought scrubs are formulated for specific skin types, or for all types. One of our favorite recipes is for a homemade scrub for oily skin that will work for all skin types (see #46). Always apply scrub in an upward and outward motion. Don't touch the eye area.

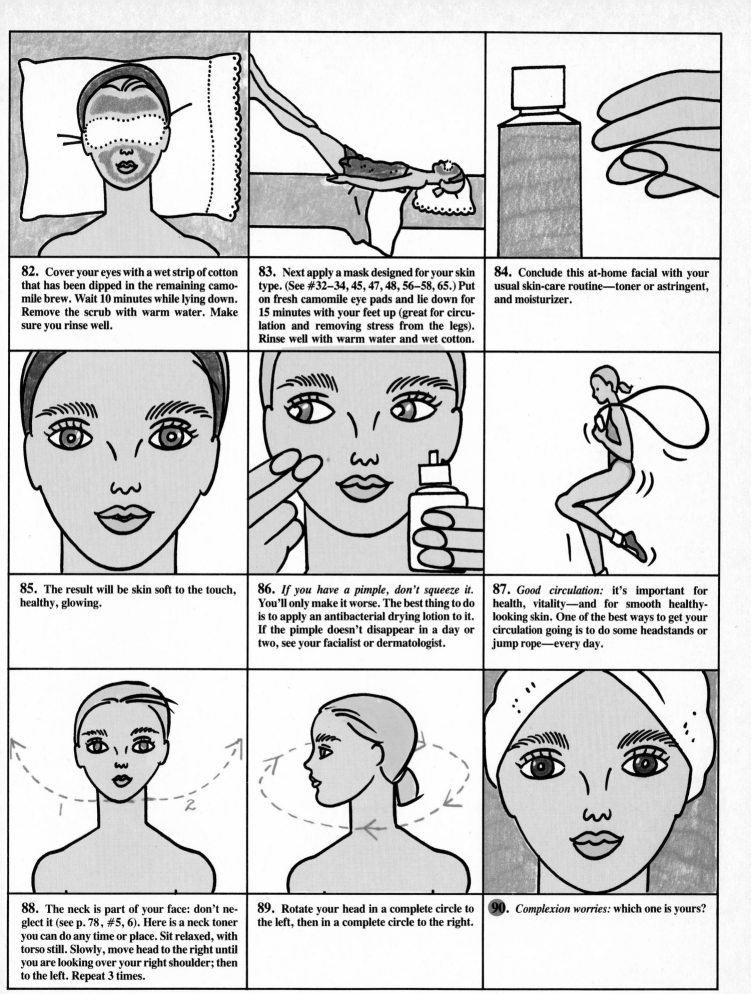

82. Cover your eyes with a wet strip of cotton that has been dipped in the remaining camomile brew. Wait 10 minutes while lying down. Remove the scrub with warm water. Make sure you rinse well.

83. Next apply a mask designed for your skin type. (See #32–34, 45, 47, 48, 56–58, 65.) Put on fresh camomile eye pads and lie down for 15 minutes with your feet up (great for circulation and removing stress from the legs). Rinse well with warm water and wet cotton.

84. Conclude this at-home facial with your usual skin-care routine—toner or astringent, and moisturizer.

85. The result will be skin soft to the touch, healthy, glowing.

86. *If you have a pimple, don't squeeze it.* You'll only make it worse. The best thing to do is to apply an antibacterial drying lotion to it. If the pimple doesn't disappear in a day or two, see your facialist or dermatologist.

87. *Good circulation:* it's important for health, vitality—and for smooth healthy-looking skin. One of the best ways to get your circulation going is to do some headstands or jump rope—every day.

88. The neck is part of your face: don't neglect it (see p. 78, #5, 6). Here is a neck toner you can do any time or place. Sit relaxed, with torso still. Slowly, move head to the right until you are looking over your right shoulder; then to the left. Repeat 3 times.

89. Rotate your head in a complete circle to the left, then in a complete circle to the right.

90. *Complexion worries:* which one is yours?

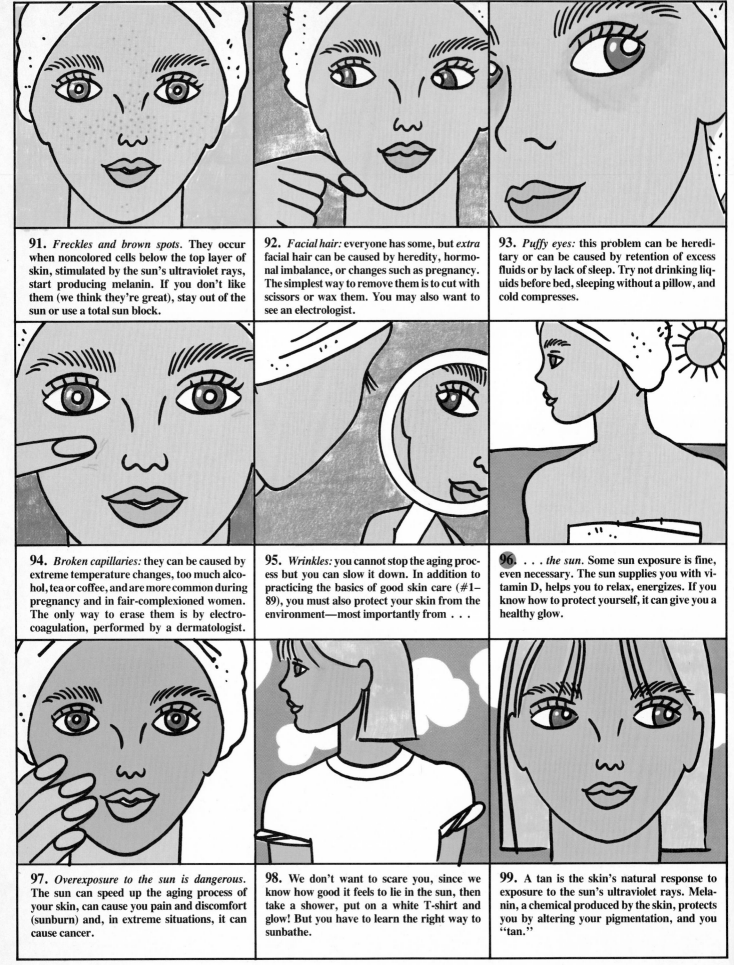

91. *Freckles and brown spots.* They occur when noncolored cells below the top layer of skin, stimulated by the sun's ultraviolet rays, start producing melanin. If you don't like them (we think they're great), stay out of the sun or use a total sun block.

92. *Facial hair:* everyone has some, but *extra* facial hair can be caused by heredity, hormonal imbalance, or changes such as pregnancy. The simplest way to remove them is to cut with scissors or wax them. You may also want to see an electrologist.

93. *Puffy eyes:* this problem can be hereditary or can be caused by retention of excess fluids or by lack of sleep. Try not drinking liquids before bed, sleeping without a pillow, and cold compresses.

94. *Broken capillaries:* they can be caused by extreme temperature changes, too much alcohol, tea or coffee, and are more common during pregnancy and in fair-complexioned women. The only way to erase them is by electrocoagulation, performed by a dermatologist.

95. *Wrinkles:* you cannot stop the aging process but you can slow it down. In addition to practicing the basics of good skin care (#1–89), you must also protect your skin from the environment—most importantly from . . .

96. . . . *the sun.* Some sun exposure is fine, even necessary. The sun supplies you with vitamin D, helps you to relax, energizes. If you know how to protect yourself, it can give you a healthy glow.

97. *Overexposure to the sun is dangerous.* The sun can speed up the aging process of your skin, can cause you pain and discomfort (sunburn) and, in extreme situations, it can cause cancer.

98. We don't want to scare you, since we know how good it feels to lie in the sun, then take a shower, put on a white T-shirt and glow! But you have to learn the right way to sunbathe.

99. A tan is the skin's natural response to exposure to the sun's ultraviolet rays. Melanin, a chemical produced by the skin, protects you by altering your pigmentation, and you "tan."

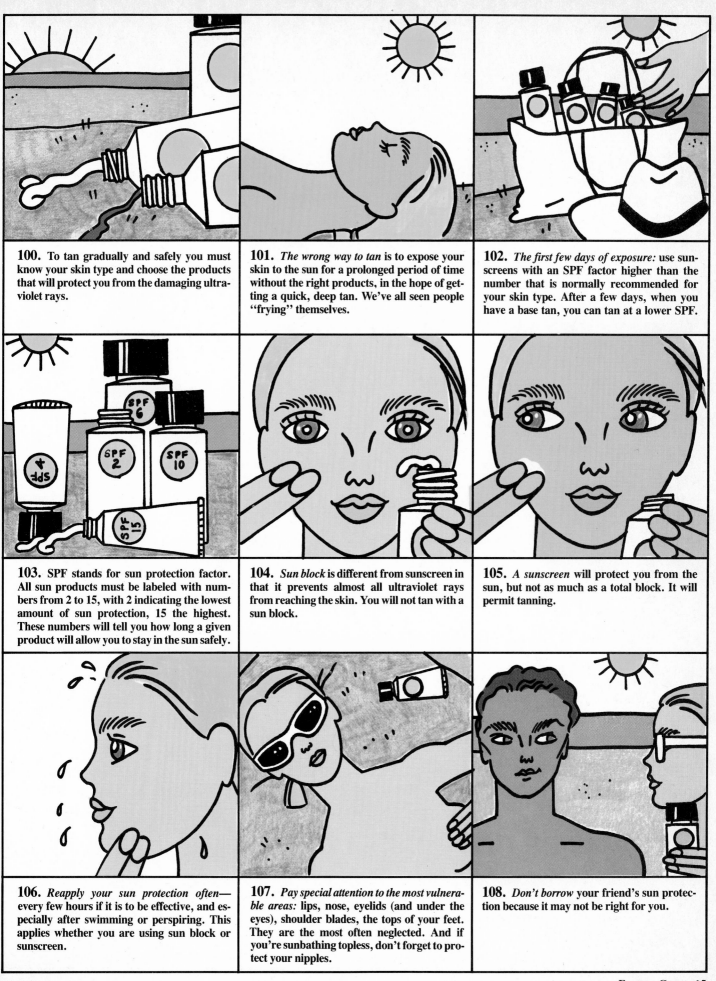

100. To tan gradually and safely you must know your skin type and choose the products that will protect you from the damaging ultraviolet rays.

101. *The wrong way to tan* is to expose your skin to the sun for a prolonged period of time without the right products, in the hope of getting a quick, deep tan. We've all seen people "frying" themselves.

102. *The first few days of exposure:* use sunscreens with an SPF factor higher than the number that is normally recommended for your skin type. After a few days, when you have a base tan, you can tan at a lower SPF.

103. SPF stands for sun protection factor. All sun products must be labeled with numbers from 2 to 15, with 2 indicating the lowest amount of sun protection, 15 the highest. These numbers will tell you how long a given product will allow you to stay in the sun safely.

104. *Sun block* is different from sunscreen in that it prevents almost all ultraviolet rays from reaching the skin. You will not tan with a sun block.

105. *A sunscreen* will protect you from the sun, but not as much as a total block. It will permit tanning.

106. *Reapply your sun protection often—* every few hours if it is to be effective, and especially after swimming or perspiring. This applies whether you are using sun block or sunscreen.

107. *Pay special attention to the most vulnerable areas:* lips, nose, eyelids (and under the eyes), shoulder blades, the tops of your feet. They are the most often neglected. And if you're sunbathing topless, don't forget to protect your nipples.

108. *Don't borrow* your friend's sun protection because it may not be right for you.

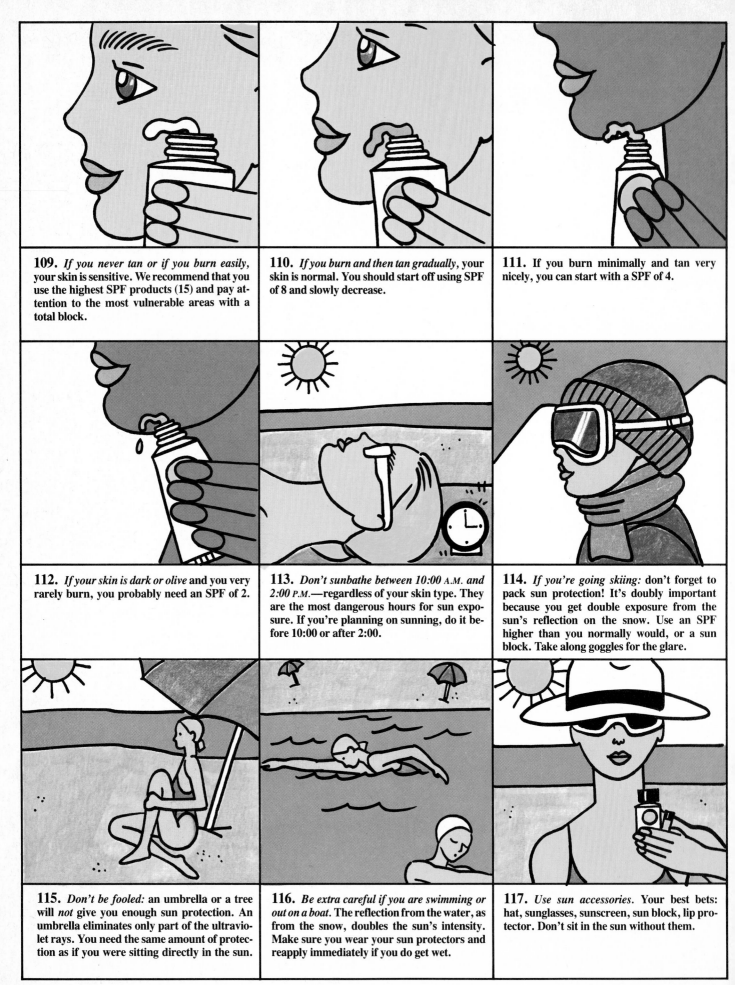

109. *If you never tan or if you burn easily,* your skin is sensitive. We recommend that you use the highest SPF products (15) and pay attention to the most vulnerable areas with a total block.

110. *If you burn and then tan gradually,* your skin is normal. You should start off using SPF of 8 and slowly decrease.

111. If you burn minimally and tan very nicely, you can start with a SPF of 4.

112. *If your skin is dark or olive* and you very rarely burn, you probably need an SPF of 2.

113. *Don't sunbathe between 10:00 A.M. and 2:00 P.M.*—regardless of your skin type. They are the most dangerous hours for sun exposure. If you're planning on sunning, do it before 10:00 or after 2:00.

114. *If you're going skiing:* don't forget to pack sun protection! It's doubly important because you get double exposure from the sun's reflection on the snow. Use an SPF higher than you normally would, or a sun block. Take along goggles for the glare.

115. *Don't be fooled:* an umbrella or a tree will *not* give you enough sun protection. An umbrella eliminates only part of the ultraviolet rays. You need the same amount of protection as if you were sitting directly in the sun.

116. *Be extra careful if you are swimming or out on a boat.* The reflection from the water, as from the snow, doubles the sun's intensity. Make sure you wear your sun protectors and reapply immediately if you do get wet.

117. *Use sun accessories.* Your best bets: hat, sunglasses, sunscreen, sun block, lip protector. Don't sit in the sun without them.

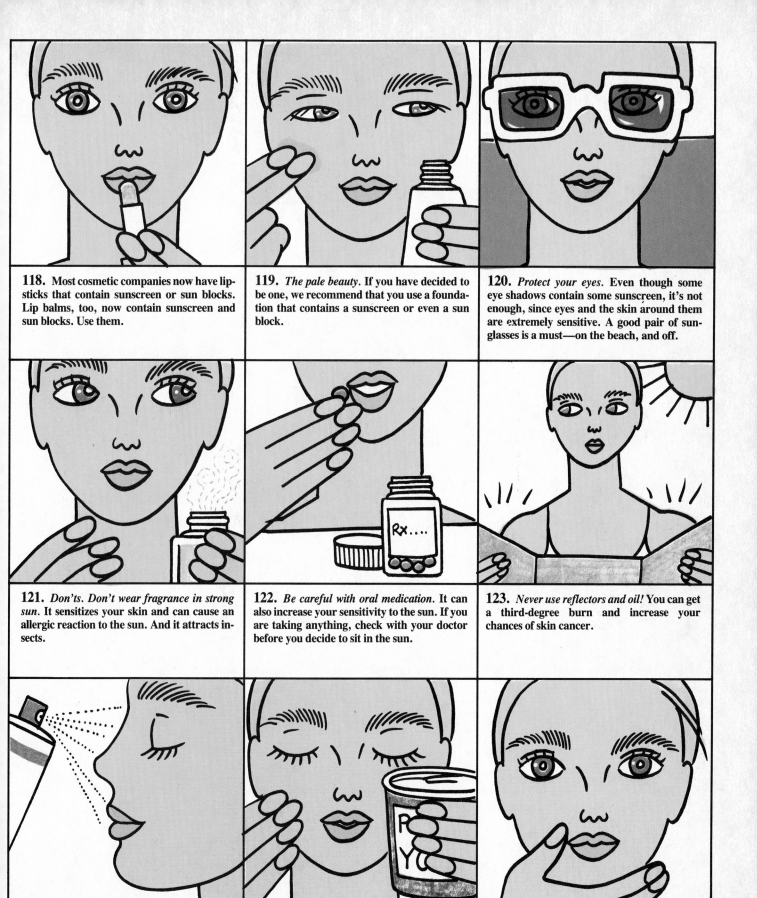

118. Most cosmetic companies now have lipsticks that contain sunscreen or sun blocks. Lip balms, too, now contain sunscreen and sun blocks. Use them.

119. *The pale beauty*. If you have decided to be one, we recommend that you use a foundation that contains a sunscreen or even a sun block.

120. *Protect your eyes*. Even though some eye shadows contain some sunscreen, it's not enough, since eyes and the skin around them are extremely sensitive. A good pair of sunglasses is a must—on the beach, and off.

121. *Don'ts. Don't wear fragrance in strong sun.* It sensitizes your skin and can cause an allergic reaction to the sun. And it attracts insects.

122. *Be careful with oral medication.* It can also increase your sensitivity to the sun. If you are taking anything, check with your doctor before you decide to sit in the sun.

123. *Never use reflectors and oil!* You can get a third-degree burn and increase your chances of skin cancer.

124. *Something extra for your face:* if your face is exposed to chlorine or salt water, we recommend that you spritz it with mineral water before you reapply your sunscreen or block.

125. *After-sun soother:* Apply a hydrating, moisturizing mask that will replenish your skin with the moisture you lost during sunbathing. The best one we know of is cold plain yogurt straight from the refrigerator.

126. *Remember—sun damage is cumulative.* It doesn't appear right away. It is never too early to discipline yourself and observe the simple rules of good basic skin care. It's up to you to prevent the preventable.

2
MAKE-UP

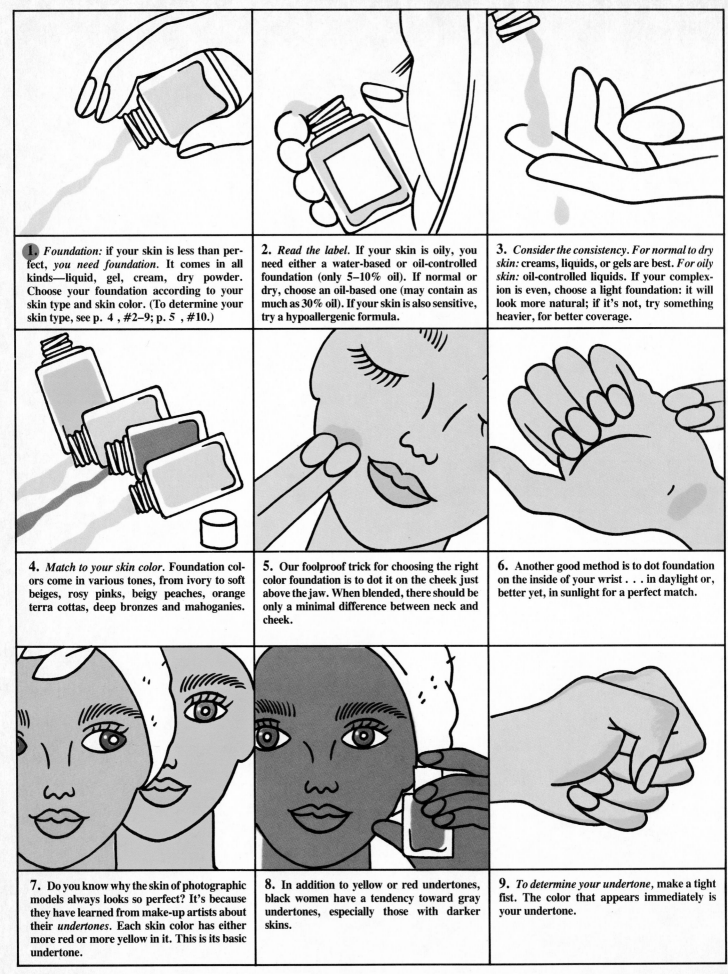

1. *Foundation:* if your skin is less than perfect, *you need foundation.* It comes in all kinds—liquid, gel, cream, dry powder. Choose your foundation according to your skin type and skin color. (To determine your skin type, see p. 4 , #2–9; p. 5 , #10.)

2. *Read the label.* If your skin is oily, you need either a water-based or oil-controlled foundation (only 5–10% oil). If normal or dry, choose an oil-based one (may contain as much as 30% oil). If your skin is also sensitive, try a hypoallergenic formula.

3. *Consider the consistency. For normal to dry skin:* creams, liquids, or gels are best. *For oily skin:* oil-controlled liquids. If your complexion is even, choose a light foundation: it will look more natural; if it's not, try something heavier, for better coverage.

4. *Match to your skin color.* Foundation colors come in various tones, from ivory to soft beiges, rosy pinks, beigy peaches, orange terra cottas, deep bronzes and mahoganies.

5. Our foolproof trick for choosing the right color foundation is to dot it on the cheek just above the jaw. When blended, there should be only a minimal difference between neck and cheek.

6. Another good method is to dot foundation on the inside of your wrist . . . in daylight or, better yet, in sunlight for a perfect match.

7. Do you know why the skin of photographic models always looks so perfect? It's because they have learned from make-up artists about their *undertones.* Each skin color has either more red or more yellow in it. This is its basic undertone.

8. In addition to yellow or red undertones, black women have a tendency toward gray undertones, especially those with darker skins.

9. *To determine your undertone,* make a tight fist. The color that appears immediately is your undertone.

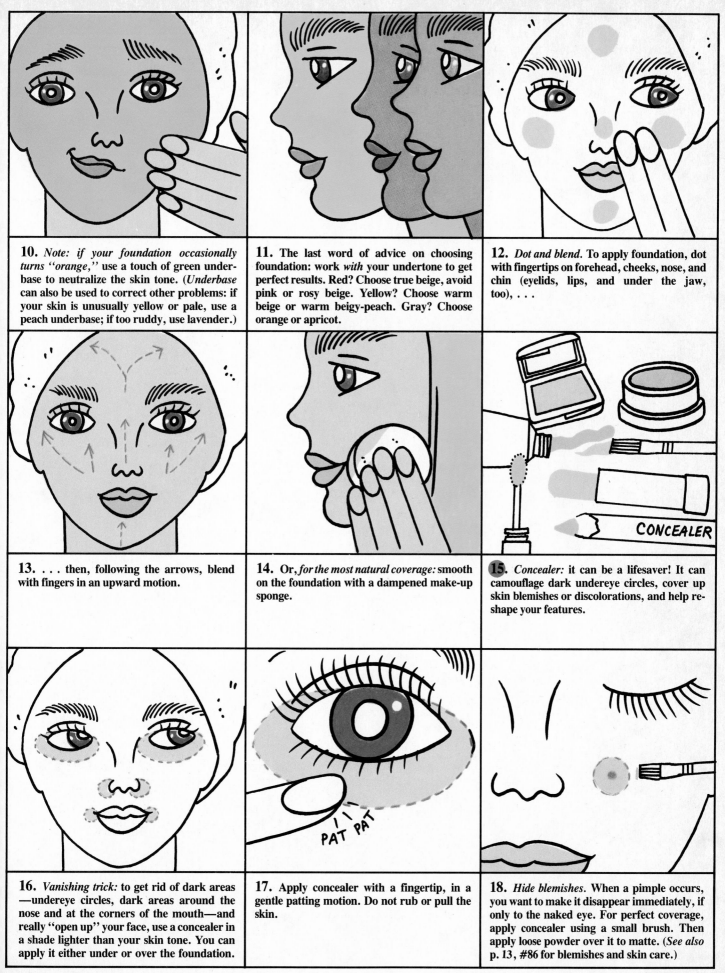

10. *Note: if your foundation occasionally turns "orange,"* use a touch of green underbase to neutralize the skin tone. (*Underbase* can also be used to correct other problems: if your skin is unusually yellow or pale, use a peach underbase; if too ruddy, use lavender.)

11. The last word of advice on choosing foundation: work *with* your undertone to get perfect results. Red? Choose true beige, avoid pink or rosy beige. Yellow? Choose warm beige or warm beigy-peach. Gray? Choose orange or apricot.

12. *Dot and blend.* To apply foundation, dot with fingertips on forehead, cheeks, nose, and chin (eyelids, lips, and under the jaw, too), . . .

13. . . . then, following the arrows, blend with fingers in an upward motion.

14. Or, *for the most natural coverage:* smooth on the foundation with a dampened make-up sponge.

15. *Concealer:* it can be a lifesaver! It can camouflage dark undereye circles, cover up skin blemishes or discolorations, and help reshape your features.

16. *Vanishing trick:* to get rid of dark areas —undereye circles, dark areas around the nose and at the corners of the mouth—and really "open up" your face, use a concealer in a shade lighter than your skin tone. You can apply it either under or over the foundation.

17. Apply concealer with a fingertip, in a gentle patting motion. Do not rub or pull the skin.

18. *Hide blemishes.* When a pimple occurs, you want to make it disappear immediately, if only to the naked eye. For perfect coverage, apply concealer using a small brush. Then apply loose powder over it to matte. (*See also* p. 13, #86 for blemishes and skin care.)

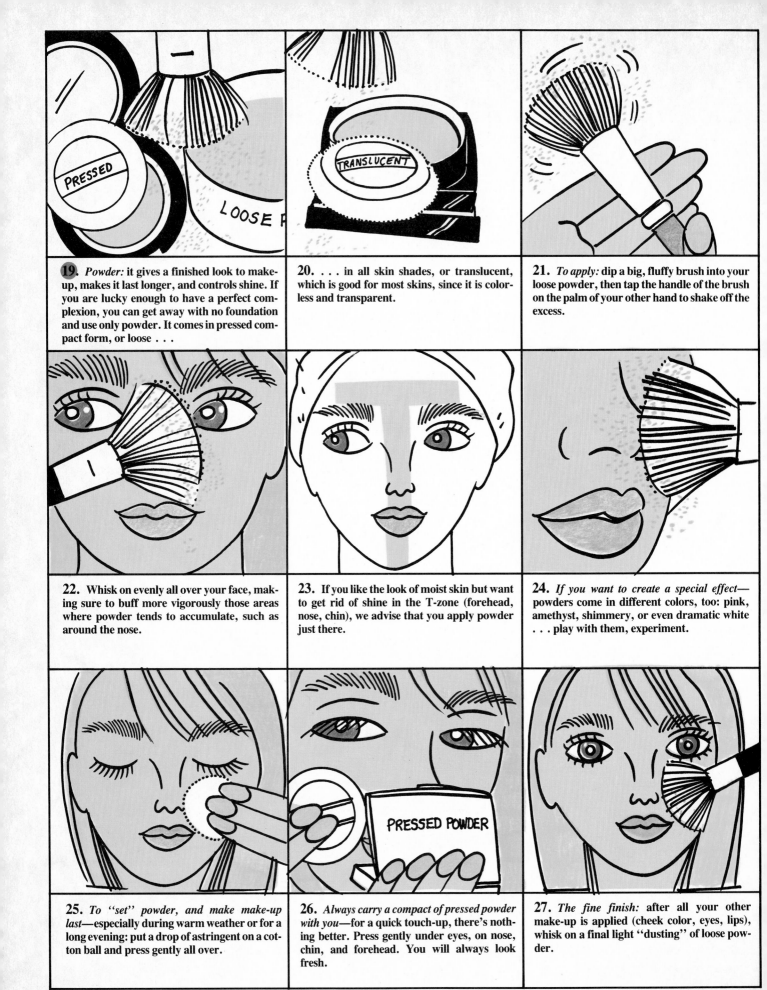

19. *Powder:* it gives a finished look to make-up, makes it last longer, and controls shine. If you are lucky enough to have a perfect complexion, you can get away with no foundation and use only powder. It comes in pressed compact form, or loose . . .

20. . . . in all skin shades, or translucent, which is good for most skins, since it is colorless and transparent.

21. *To apply:* dip a big, fluffy brush into your loose powder, then tap the handle of the brush on the palm of your other hand to shake off the excess.

22. Whisk on evenly all over your face, making sure to buff more vigorously those areas where powder tends to accumulate, such as around the nose.

23. If you like the look of moist skin but want to get rid of shine in the T-zone (forehead, nose, chin), we advise that you apply powder just there.

24. *If you want to create a special effect—*powders come in different colors, too: pink, amethyst, shimmery, or even dramatic white . . . play with them, experiment.

25. *To "set" powder, and make make-up last—*especially during warm weather or for a long evening: put a drop of astringent on a cotton ball and press gently all over.

26. *Always carry a compact of pressed powder with you—*for a quick touch-up, there's nothing better. Press gently under eyes, on nose, chin, and forehead. You will always look fresh.

27. *The fine finish:* after all your other make-up is applied (cheek color, eyes, lips), whisk on a final light "dusting" of loose powder.

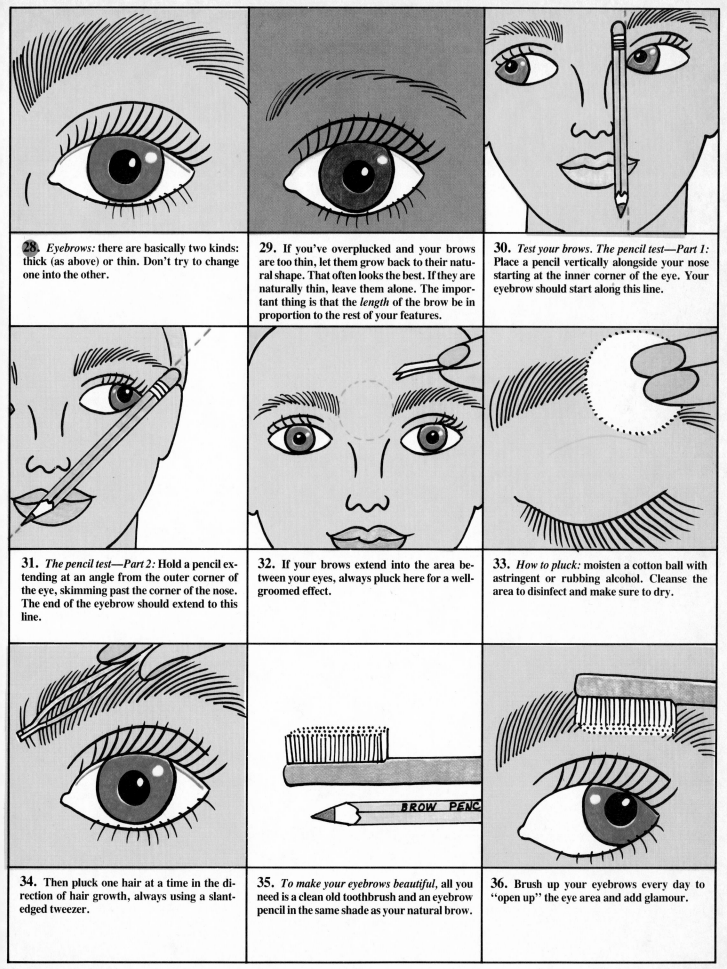

28. *Eyebrows:* there are basically two kinds: thick (as above) or thin. Don't try to change one into the other.

29. If you've overplucked and your brows are too thin, let them grow back to their natural shape. That often looks the best. If they are naturally thin, leave them alone. The important thing is that the *length* of the brow be in proportion to the rest of your features.

30. *Test your brows. The pencil test—Part 1:* Place a pencil vertically alongside your nose starting at the inner corner of the eye. Your eyebrow should start along this line.

31. *The pencil test—Part 2:* Hold a pencil extending at an angle from the outer corner of the eye, skimming past the corner of the nose. The end of the eyebrow should extend to this line.

32. If your brows extend into the area between your eyes, always pluck here for a well-groomed effect.

33. *How to pluck:* moisten a cotton ball with astringent or rubbing alcohol. Cleanse the area to disinfect and make sure to dry.

34. Then pluck one hair at a time in the direction of hair growth, always using a slant-edged tweezer.

35. *To make your eyebrows beautiful,* all you need is a clean old toothbrush and an eyebrow pencil in the same shade as your natural brow.

36. Brush up your eyebrows every day to "open up" the eye area and add glamour.

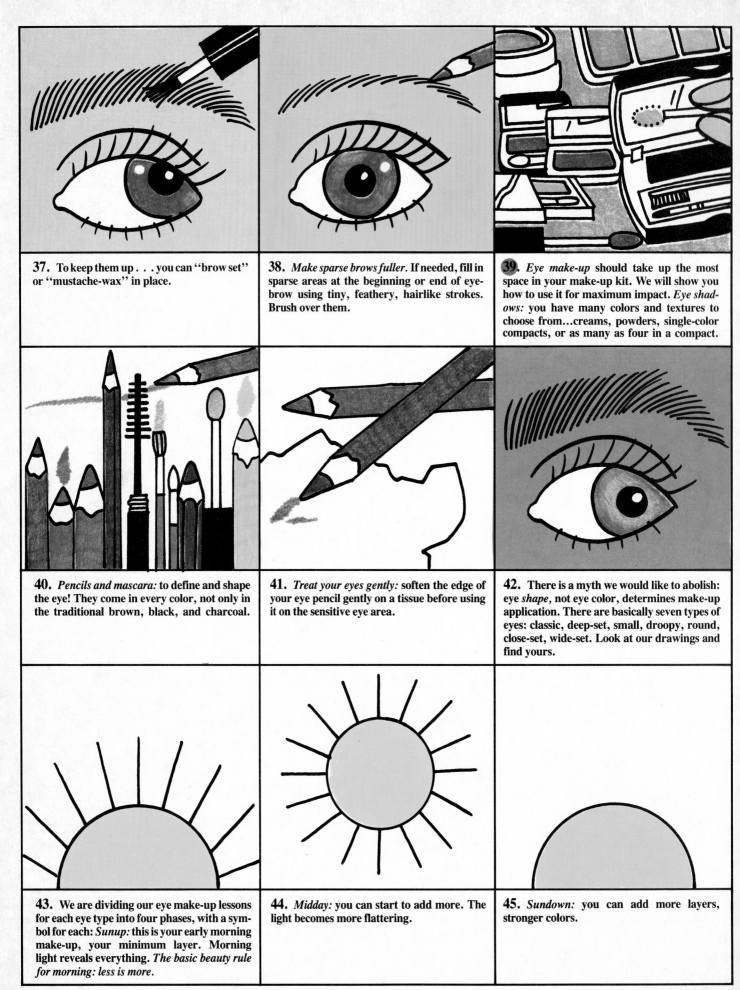

37. To keep them up . . . you can "brow set" or "mustache-wax" in place.

38. *Make sparse brows fuller.* If needed, fill in sparse areas at the beginning or end of eyebrow using tiny, feathery, hairlike strokes. Brush over them.

39. *Eye make-up* should take up the most space in your make-up kit. We will show you how to use it for maximum impact. *Eye shadows:* you have many colors and textures to choose from...creams, powders, single-color compacts, or as many as four in a compact.

40. *Pencils and mascara:* to define and shape the eye! They come in every color, not only in the traditional brown, black, and charcoal.

41. *Treat your eyes gently:* soften the edge of your eye pencil gently on a tissue before using it on the sensitive eye area.

42. There is a myth we would like to abolish: eye *shape*, not eye color, determines make-up application. There are basically seven types of eyes: classic, deep-set, small, droopy, round, close-set, wide-set. Look at our drawings and find yours.

43. We are dividing our eye make-up lessons for each eye type into four phases, with a symbol for each: *Sunup:* this is your early morning make-up, your minimum layer. Morning light reveals everything. *The basic beauty rule for morning: less is more.*

44. *Midday:* you can start to add more. The light becomes more flattering.

45. *Sundown:* you can add more layers, stronger colors.

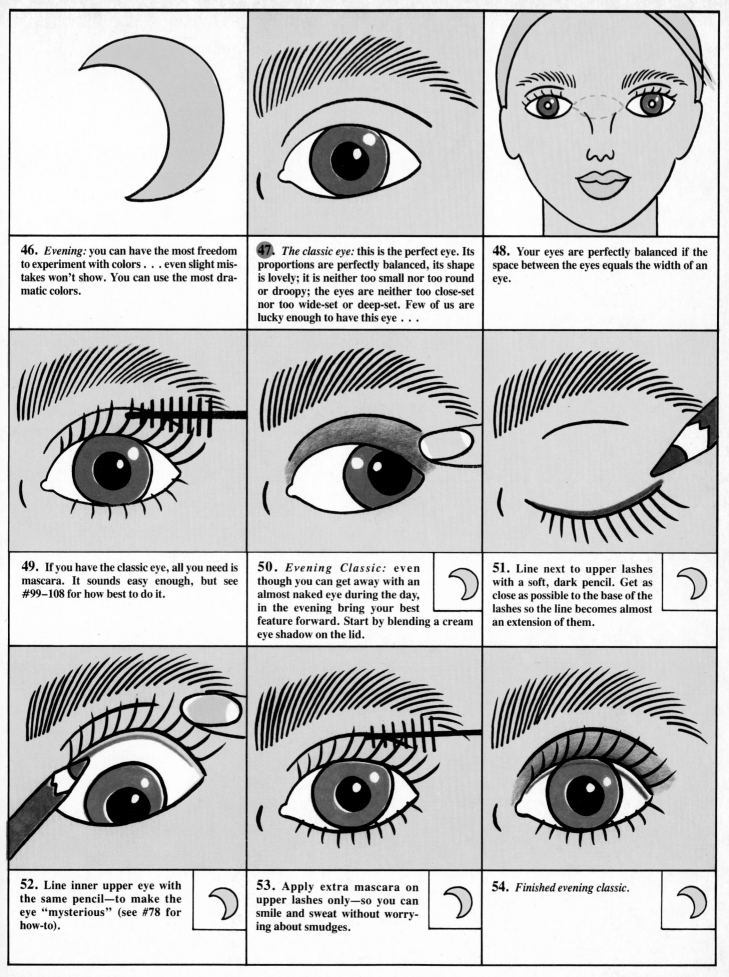

46. *Evening:* you can have the most freedom to experiment with colors . . . even slight mistakes won't show. You can use the most dramatic colors.

47. *The classic eye:* this is the perfect eye. Its proportions are perfectly balanced, its shape is lovely; it is neither too small nor too round or droopy; the eyes are neither too close-set nor too wide-set or deep-set. Few of us are lucky enough to have this eye . . .

48. Your eyes are perfectly balanced if the space between the eyes equals the width of an eye.

49. If you have the classic eye, all you need is mascara. It sounds easy enough, but see #99–108 for how best to do it.

50. *Evening Classic:* even though you can get away with an almost naked eye during the day, in the evening bring your best feature forward. Start by blending a cream eye shadow on the lid.

51. Line next to upper lashes with a soft, dark pencil. Get as close as possible to the base of the lashes so the line becomes almost an extension of them.

52. Line inner upper eye with the same pencil—to make the eye "mysterious" (see #78 for how-to).

53. Apply extra mascara on upper lashes only—so you can smile and sweat without worrying about smudges.

54. *Finished evening classic.*

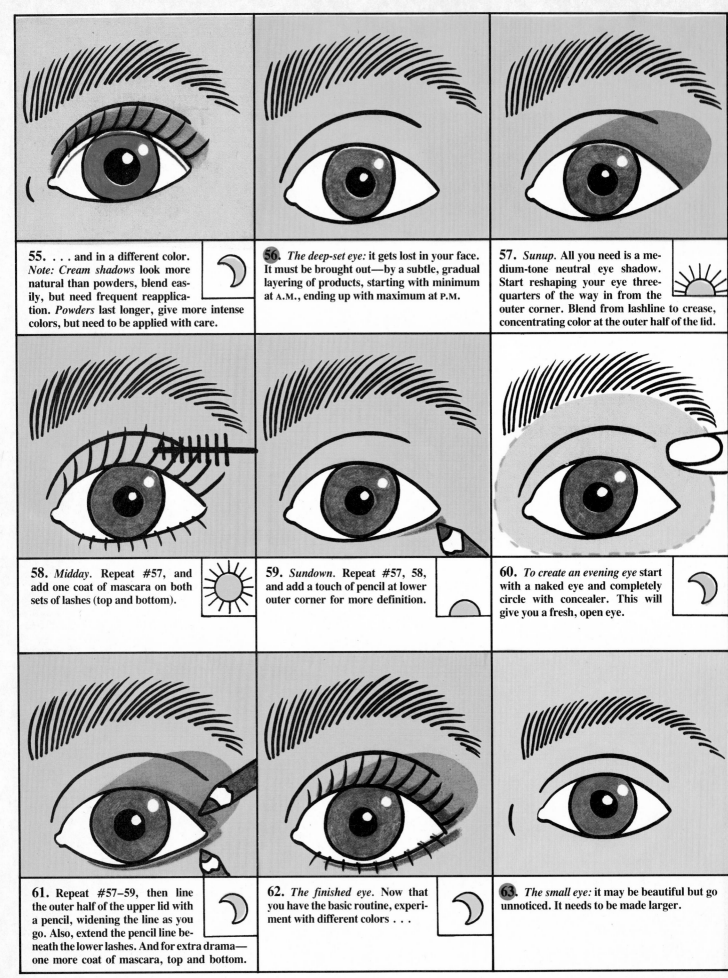

55. . . . and in a different color. *Note: Cream shadows* look more natural than powders, blend easily, but need frequent reapplication. *Powders* last longer, give more intense colors, but need to be applied with care.

56. *The deep-set eye:* it gets lost in your face. It must be brought out—by a subtle, gradual layering of products, starting with minimum at A.M., ending up with maximum at P.M.

57. *Sunup.* All you need is a medium-tone neutral eye shadow. Start reshaping your eye three-quarters of the way in from the outer corner. Blend from lashline to crease, concentrating color at the outer half of the lid.

58. *Midday.* Repeat #57, and add one coat of mascara on both sets of lashes (top and bottom).

59. *Sundown.* Repeat #57, 58, and add a touch of pencil at lower outer corner for more definition.

60. *To create an evening eye* start with a naked eye and completely circle with concealer. This will give you a fresh, open eye.

61. Repeat #57–59, then line the outer half of the upper lid with a pencil, widening the line as you go. Also, extend the pencil line beneath the lower lashes. And for extra drama— one more coat of mascara, top and bottom.

62. *The finished eye.* Now that you have the basic routine, experiment with different colors . . .

63. *The small eye:* it may be beautiful but go unnoticed. It needs to be made larger.

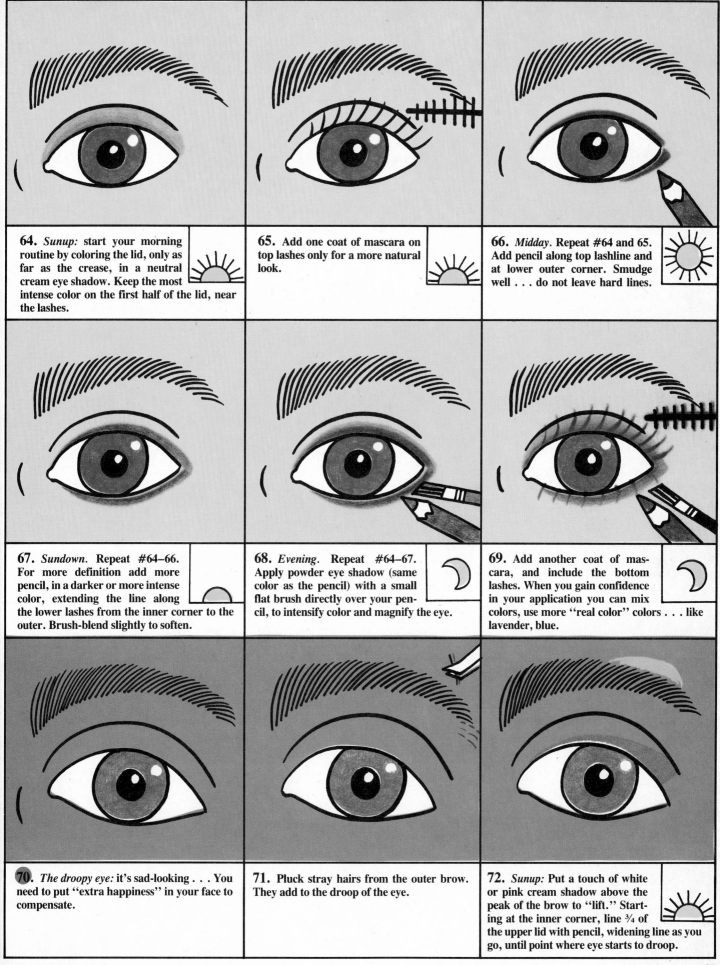

64. *Sunup:* start your morning routine by coloring the lid, only as far as the crease, in a neutral cream eye shadow. Keep the most intense color on the first half of the lid, near the lashes.

65. Add one coat of mascara on top lashes only for a more natural look.

66. *Midday.* Repeat #64 and 65. Add pencil along top lashline and at lower outer corner. Smudge well . . . do not leave hard lines.

67. *Sundown.* Repeat #64–66. For more definition add more pencil, in a darker or more intense color, extending the line along the lower lashes from the inner corner to the outer. Brush-blend slightly to soften.

68. *Evening.* Repeat #64–67. Apply powder eye shadow (same color as the pencil) with a small flat brush directly over your pencil, to intensify color and magnify the eye.

69. Add another coat of mascara, and include the bottom lashes. When you gain confidence in your application you can mix colors, use more "real color" colors . . . like lavender, blue.

70. *The droopy eye:* it's sad-looking . . . You need to put "extra happiness" in your face to compensate.

71. Pluck stray hairs from the outer brow. They add to the droop of the eye.

72. *Sunup:* Put a touch of white or pink cream shadow above the peak of the brow to "lift." Starting at the inner corner, line ¾ of the upper lid with pencil, widening line as you go, until point where eye starts to droop.

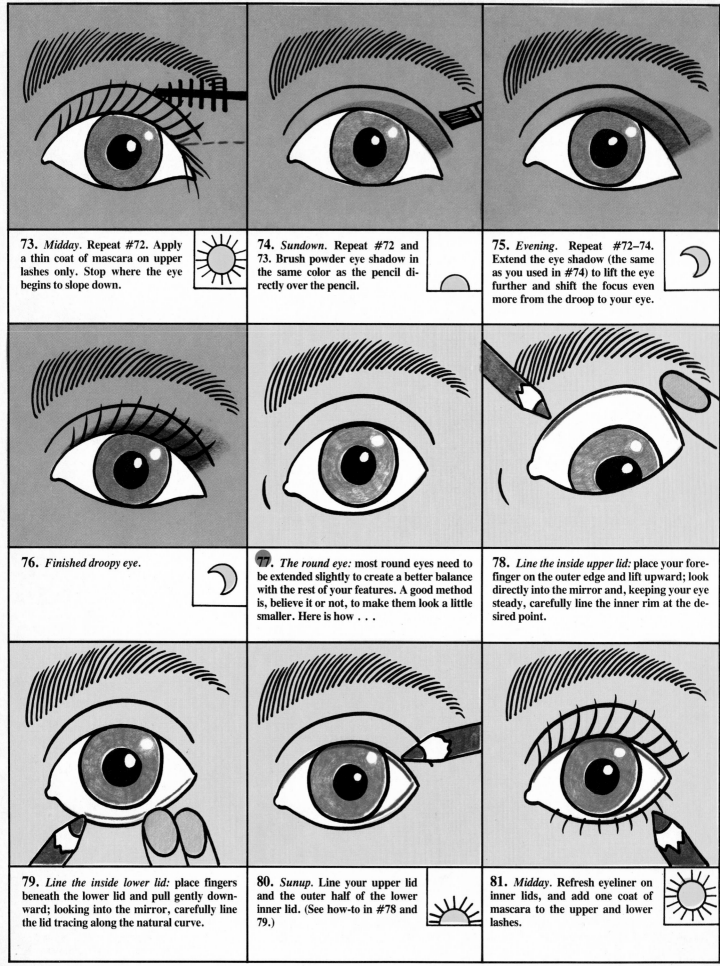

73. *Midday*. Repeat #72. Apply a thin coat of mascara on upper lashes only. Stop where the eye begins to slope down.

74. *Sundown*. Repeat #72 and 73. Brush powder eye shadow in the same color as the pencil directly over the pencil.

75. *Evening*. Repeat #72–74. Extend the eye shadow (the same as you used in #74) to lift the eye further and shift the focus even more from the droop to your eye.

76. *Finished droopy eye.*

77. *The round eye:* most round eyes need to be extended slightly to create a better balance with the rest of your features. A good method is, believe it or not, to make them look a little smaller. Here is how . . .

78. *Line the inside upper lid:* place your forefinger on the outer edge and lift upward; look directly into the mirror and, keeping your eye steady, carefully line the inner rim at the desired point.

79. *Line the inside lower lid:* place fingers beneath the lower lid and pull gently downward; looking into the mirror, carefully line the lid tracing along the natural curve.

80. *Sunup*. Line your upper lid and the outer half of the lower inner lid. (See how-to in #78 and 79.)

81. *Midday*. Refresh eyeliner on inner lids, and add one coat of mascara to the upper and lower lashes.

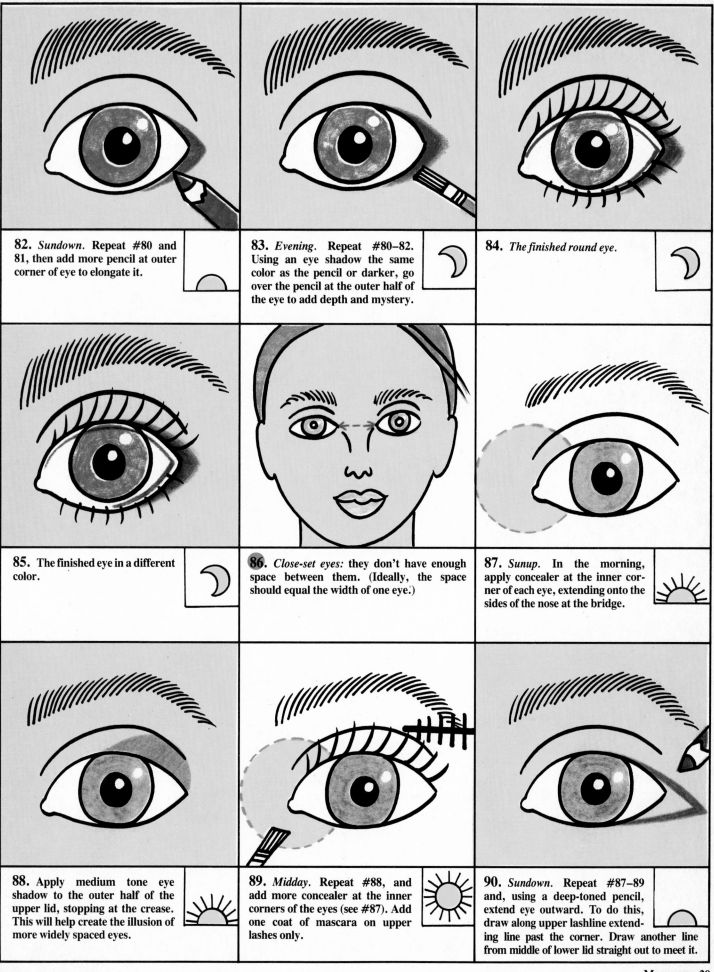

82. *Sundown.* Repeat #80 and 81, then add more pencil at outer corner of eye to elongate it.

83. *Evening.* **Repeat #80–82. Using an eye shadow the same color as the pencil or darker, go over the pencil at the outer half of the eye to add depth and mystery.**

84. *The finished round eye.*

85. The finished eye in a different color.

86. *Close-set eyes:* they don't have enough space between them. (Ideally, the space should equal the width of one eye.)

87. *Sunup.* In the morning, apply concealer at the inner corner of each eye, extending onto the sides of the nose at the bridge.

88. Apply medium tone eye shadow to the outer half of the upper lid, stopping at the crease. This will help create the illusion of more widely spaced eyes.

89. *Midday.* Repeat #88, and add more concealer at the inner corners of the eyes (see #87). Add one coat of mascara on upper lashes only.

90. *Sundown.* Repeat #87–89 and, using a deep-toned pencil, extend eye outward. To do this, draw along upper lashline extending line past the corner. Draw another line from middle of lower lid straight out to meet it.

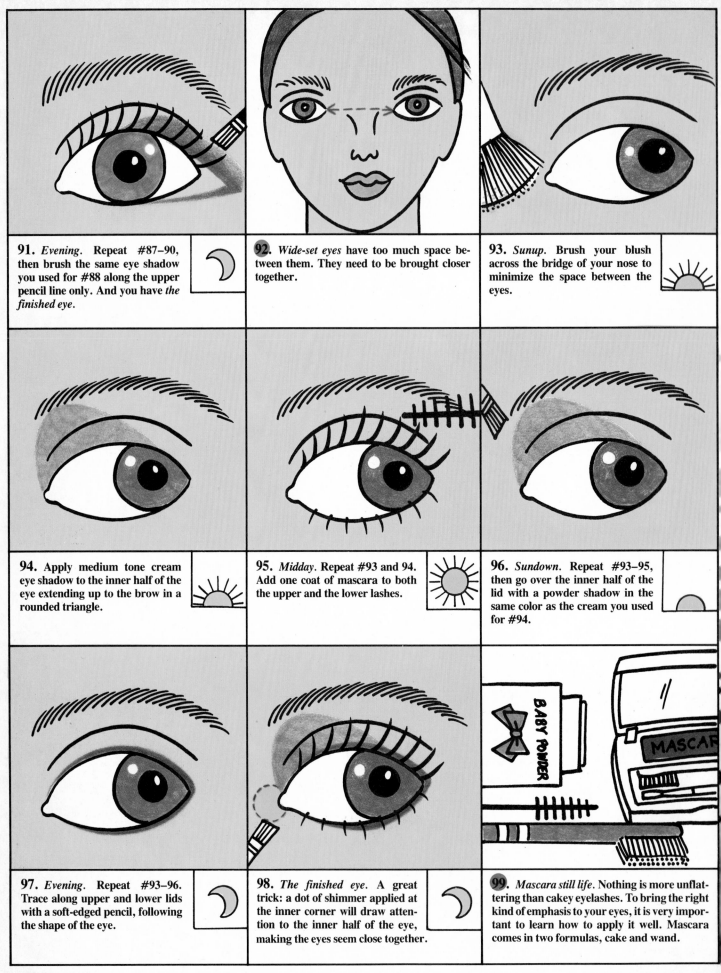

91. *Evening*. Repeat #87–90, then brush the same eye shadow you used for #88 along the upper pencil line only. And you have *the finished eye*.

92. *Wide-set eyes* have too much space between them. They need to be brought closer together.

93. *Sunup*. Brush your blush across the bridge of your nose to minimize the space between the eyes.

94. Apply medium tone cream eye shadow to the inner half of the eye extending up to the brow in a rounded triangle.

95. *Midday*. Repeat #93 and 94. Add one coat of mascara to both the upper and the lower lashes.

96. *Sundown*. Repeat #93–95, then go over the inner half of the lid with a powder shadow in the same color as the cream you used for #94.

97. *Evening*. Repeat #93–96. Trace along upper and lower lids with a soft-edged pencil, following the shape of the eye.

98. *The finished eye*. A great trick: a dot of shimmer applied at the inner corner will draw attention to the inner half of the eye, making the eyes seem close together.

99. *Mascara still life*. Nothing is more unflattering than cakey eyelashes. To bring the right kind of emphasis to your eyes, it is very important to learn how to apply it well. Mascara comes in two formulas, cake and wand.

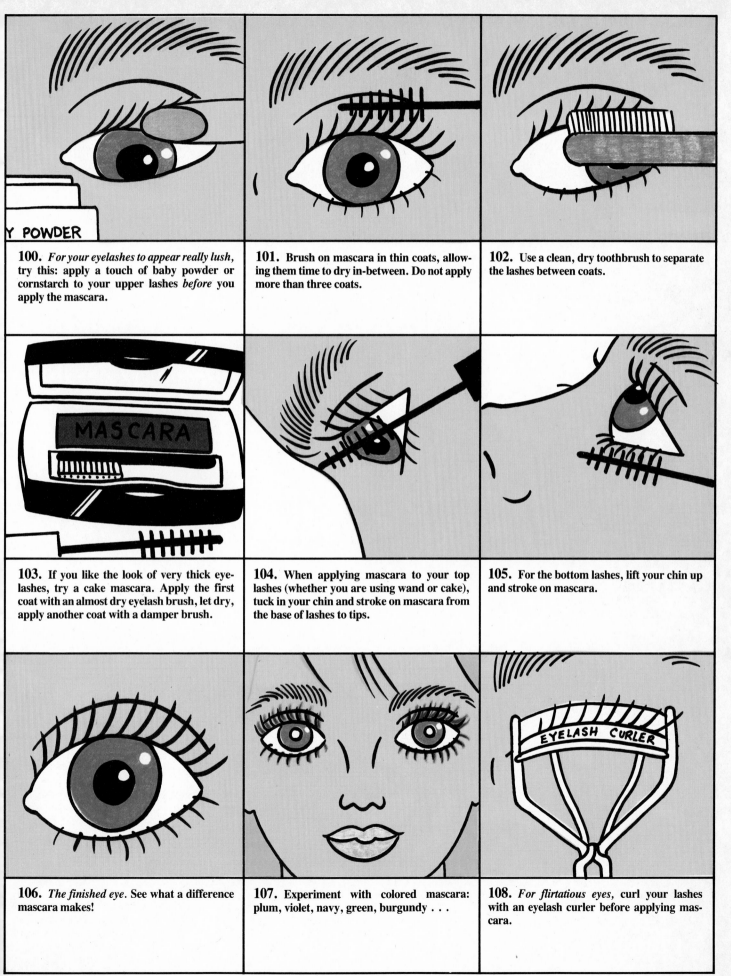

100. *For your eyelashes to appear really lush,* try this: apply a touch of baby powder or cornstarch to your upper lashes *before* you apply the mascara.

101. Brush on mascara in thin coats, allowing them time to dry in-between. Do not apply more than three coats.

102. Use a clean, dry toothbrush to separate the lashes between coats.

103. If you like the look of very thick eyelashes, try a cake mascara. Apply the first coat with an almost dry eyelash brush, let dry, apply another coat with a damper brush.

104. When applying mascara to your top lashes (whether you are using wand or cake), tuck in your chin and stroke on mascara from the base of lashes to tips.

105. For the bottom lashes, lift your chin up and stroke on mascara.

106. *The finished eye.* See what a difference mascara makes!

107. Experiment with colored mascara: plum, violet, navy, green, burgundy . . .

108. *For flirtatious eyes,* curl your lashes with an eyelash curler before applying mascara.

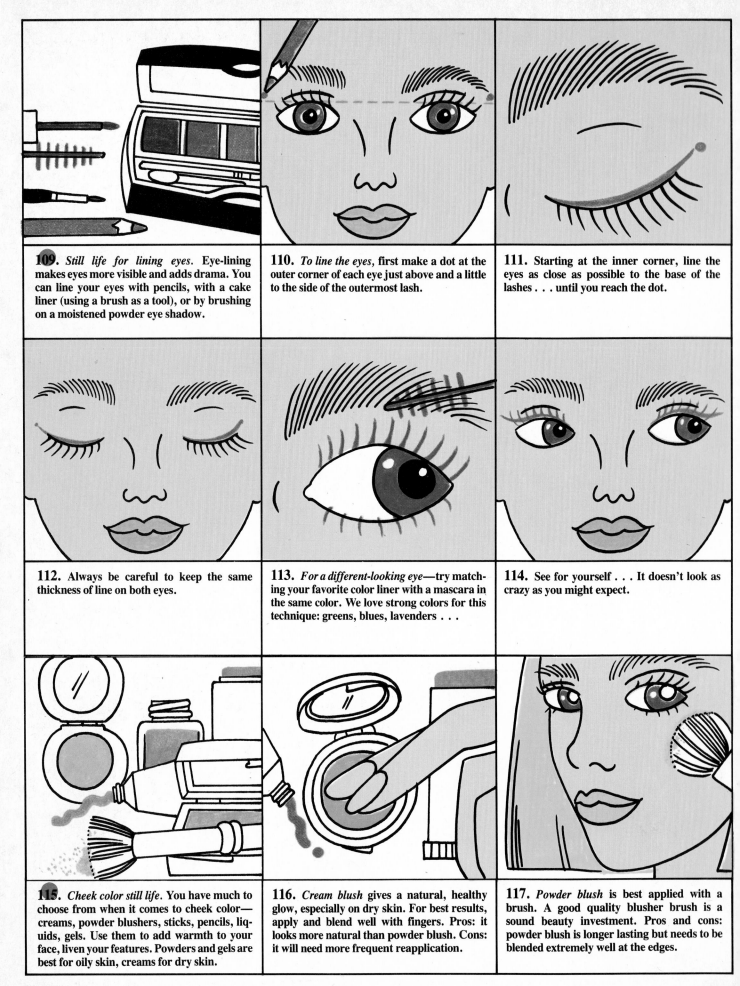

109. *Still life for lining eyes.* Eye-lining makes eyes more visible and adds drama. You can line your eyes with pencils, with a cake liner (using a brush as a tool), or by brushing on a moistened powder eye shadow.

110. *To line the eyes,* first make a dot at the outer corner of each eye just above and a little to the side of the outermost lash.

111. Starting at the inner corner, line the eyes as close as possible to the base of the lashes . . . until you reach the dot.

112. Always be careful to keep the same thickness of line on both eyes.

113. *For a different-looking eye*—try matching your favorite color liner with a mascara in the same color. We love strong colors for this technique: greens, blues, lavenders . . .

114. See for yourself . . . It doesn't look as crazy as you might expect.

115. *Cheek color still life.* You have much to choose from when it comes to cheek color—creams, powder blushers, sticks, pencils, liquids, gels. Use them to add warmth to your face, liven your features. Powders and gels are best for oily skin, creams for dry skin.

116. *Cream blush* gives a natural, healthy glow, especially on dry skin. For best results, apply and blend well with fingers. Pros: it looks more natural than powder blush. Cons: it will need more frequent reapplication.

117. *Powder blush* is best applied with a brush. A good quality blusher brush is a sound beauty investment. Pros and cons: powder blush is longer lasting but needs to be blended extremely well at the edges.

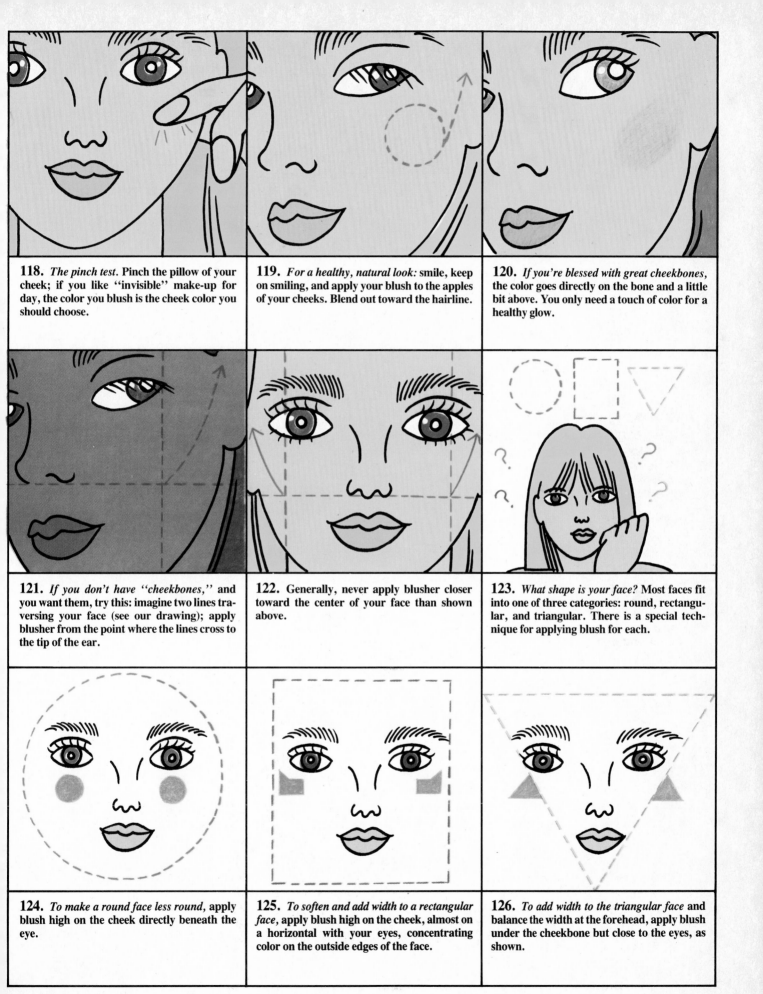

118. *The pinch test.* Pinch the pillow of your cheek; if you like "invisible" make-up for day, the color you blush is the cheek color you should choose.

119. *For a healthy, natural look:* smile, keep on smiling, and apply your blush to the apples of your cheeks. Blend out toward the hairline.

120. *If you're blessed with great cheekbones,* the color goes directly on the bone and a little bit above. You only need a touch of color for a healthy glow.

121. *If you don't have "cheekbones,"* and you want them, try this: imagine two lines traversing your face (see our drawing); apply blusher from the point where the lines cross to the tip of the ear.

122. Generally, never apply blusher closer toward the center of your face than shown above.

123. *What shape is your face?* Most faces fit into one of three categories: round, rectangular, and triangular. There is a special technique for applying blush for each.

124. *To make a round face less round,* apply blush high on the cheek directly beneath the eye.

125. *To soften and add width to a rectangular face,* apply blush high on the cheek, almost on a horizontal with your eyes, concentrating color on the outside edges of the face.

126. *To add width to the triangular face* and balance the width at the forehead, apply blush under the cheekbone but close to the eyes, as shown.

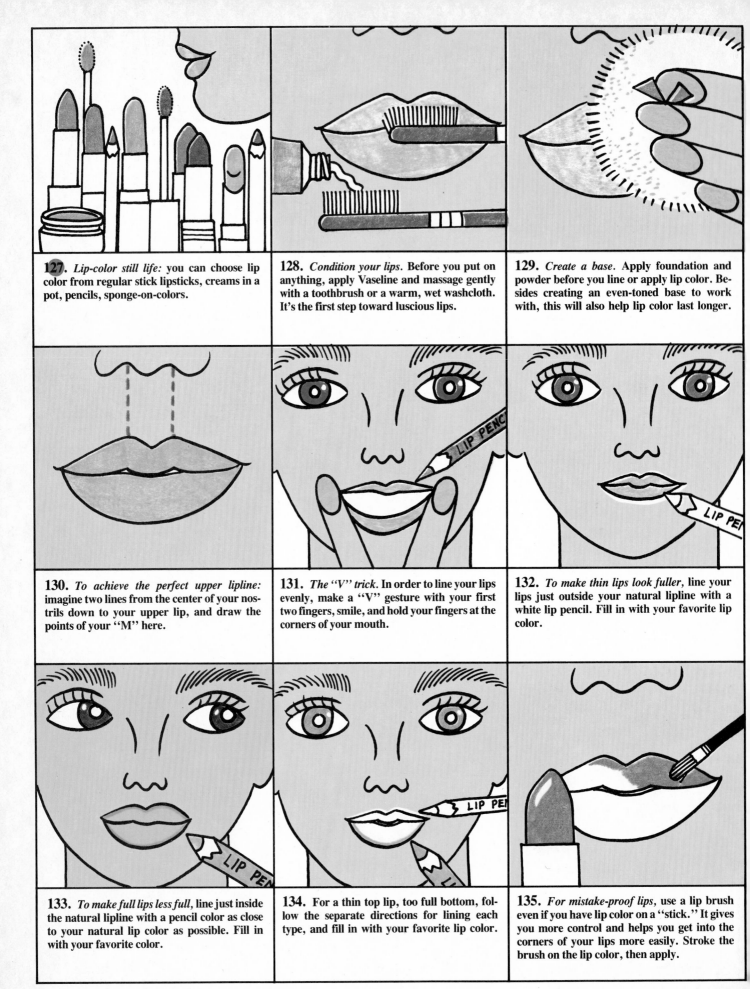

127. *Lip-color still life:* you can choose lip color from regular stick lipsticks, creams in a pot, pencils, sponge-on-colors.

128. *Condition your lips.* Before you put on anything, apply Vaseline and massage gently with a toothbrush or a warm, wet washcloth. It's the first step toward luscious lips.

129. *Create a base.* Apply foundation and powder before you line or apply lip color. Besides creating an even-toned base to work with, this will also help lip color last longer.

130. *To achieve the perfect upper lipline:* imagine two lines from the center of your nostrils down to your upper lip, and draw the points of your "M" here.

131. *The "V" trick.* In order to line your lips evenly, make a "V" gesture with your first two fingers, smile, and hold your fingers at the corners of your mouth.

132. *To make thin lips look fuller,* line your lips just outside your natural lipline with a white lip pencil. Fill in with your favorite lip color.

133. *To make full lips less full,* line just inside the natural lipline with a pencil color as close to your natural lip color as possible. Fill in with your favorite color.

134. For a thin top lip, too full bottom, follow the separate directions for lining each type, and fill in with your favorite lip color.

135. *For mistake-proof lips,* use a lip brush even if you have lip color on a "stick." It gives you more control and helps you get into the corners of your lips more easily. Stroke the brush on the lip color, then apply.

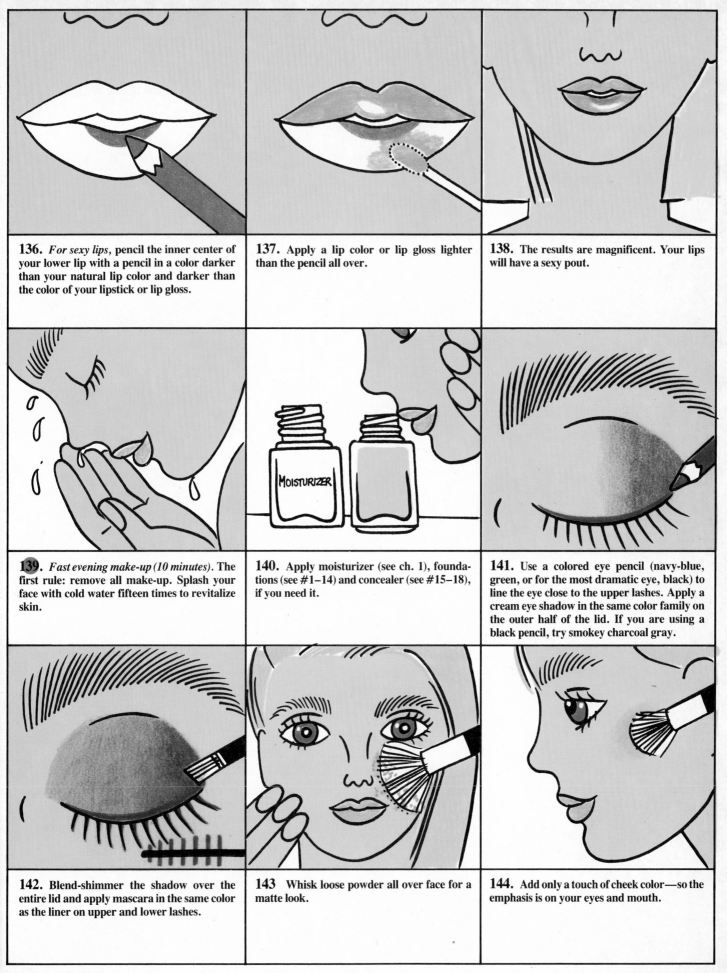

136. *For sexy lips,* pencil the inner center of your lower lip with a pencil in a color darker than your natural lip color and darker than the color of your lipstick or lip gloss.

137. Apply a lip color or lip gloss lighter than the pencil all over.

138. The results are magnificent. Your lips will have a sexy pout.

139. *Fast evening make-up (10 minutes).* The first rule: remove all make-up. Splash your face with cold water fifteen times to revitalize skin.

140. Apply moisturizer (see ch. 1), foundations (see #1–14) and concealer (see #15–18), if you need it.

141. Use a colored eye pencil (navy-blue, green, or for the most dramatic eye, black) to line the eye close to the upper lashes. Apply a cream eye shadow in the same color family on the outer half of the lid. If you are using a black pencil, try smokey charcoal gray.

142. Blend-shimmer the shadow over the entire lid and apply mascara in the same color as the liner on upper and lower lashes.

143 Whisk loose powder all over face for a matte look.

144. Add only a touch of cheek color—so the emphasis is on your eyes and mouth.

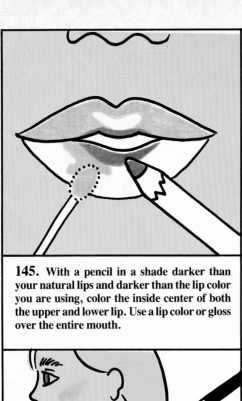

145. With a pencil in a shade darker than your natural lips and darker than the lip color you are using, color the inside center of both the upper and lower lip. Use a lip color or gloss over the entire mouth.

146. Whisk on and buff a body powder all over your exposed beauty zones—neck, shoulders, décolletage.

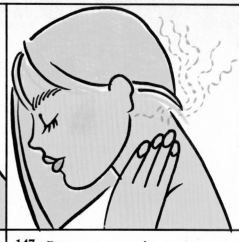

147. *Fragrance*—on pulse spots: ears, wrists, behind the knees, on décolletage, backbone, nape of neck.

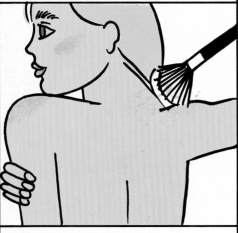

148. *For a special effect:* shimmery powders . . . on cheeks, body, lips, for sheen.

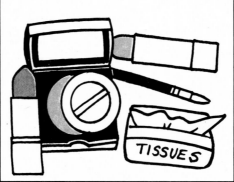

149. *The evening emergency kit,* to carry with you: lipstick, concealer, small compact pressed powder, tissues.

150. *Summer make-up:* as for morning make-up, less is more. The basic rule is: a touch of color everywhere for a vital, healthy look.

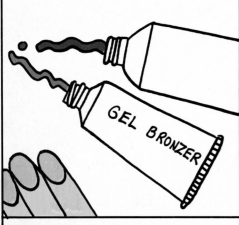

151. Assuming you have just a little bit of a healthy tan, you only need a gel bronzer to get your skin glowing. Give your skin a vacation from foundation.

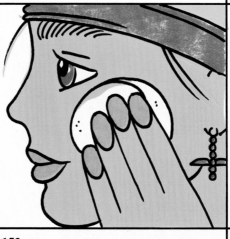

152. To get the thinnest, most even and natural application of gel, apply and blend it with a damp sponge.

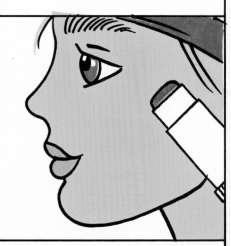

153. If you feel better with a little bit more color, use a stick cream cheek color in addition to the bronzer.

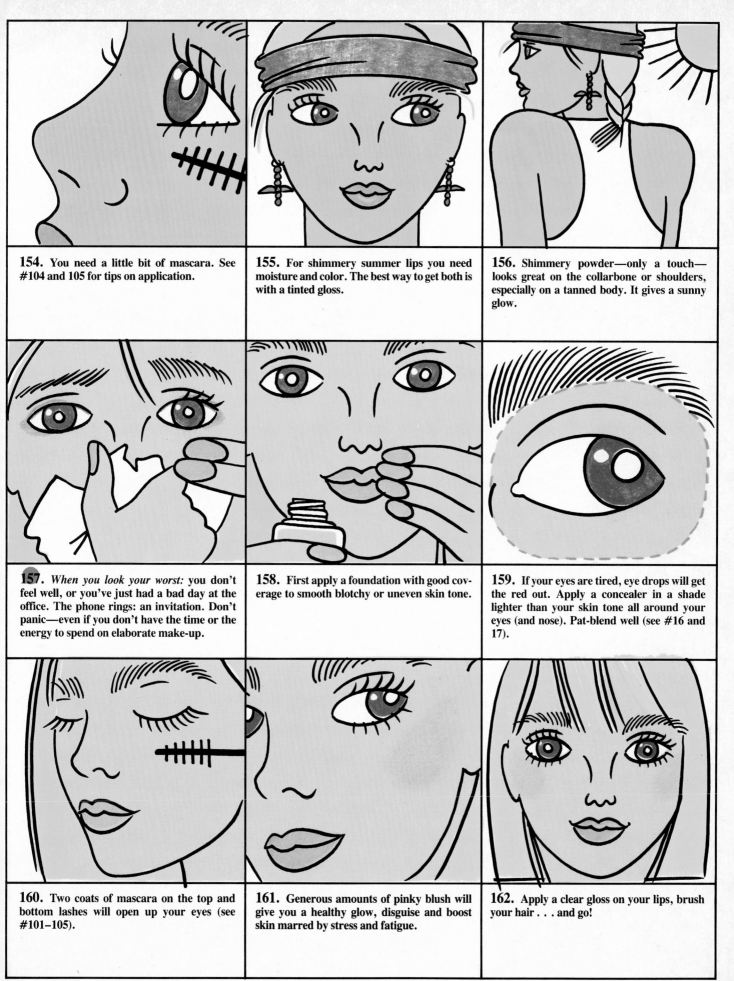

154. You need a little bit of mascara. See #104 and 105 for tips on application.

155. For shimmery summer lips you need moisture and color. The best way to get both is with a tinted gloss.

156. Shimmery powder—only a touch—looks great on the collarbone or shoulders, especially on a tanned body. It gives a sunny glow.

157. *When you look your worst:* you don't feel well, or you've just had a bad day at the office. The phone rings: an invitation. Don't panic—even if you don't have the time or the energy to spend on elaborate make-up.

158. First apply a foundation with good coverage to smooth blotchy or uneven skin tone.

159. If your eyes are tired, eye drops will get the red out. Apply a concealer in a shade lighter than your skin tone all around your eyes (and nose). Pat-blend well (see #16 and 17).

160. Two coats of mascara on the top and bottom lashes will open up your eyes (see #101–105).

161. Generous amounts of pinky blush will give you a healthy glow, disguise and boost skin marred by stress and fatigue.

162. Apply a clear gloss on your lips, brush your hair . . . and go!

3
HAIR CARE

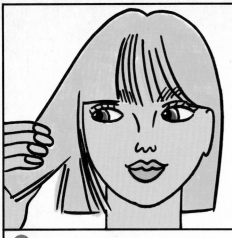

1. *Get to know your hair*. It's the next step, now that you know the type of skin you have, how to care for it, and how to make the most of it with make-up techniques.

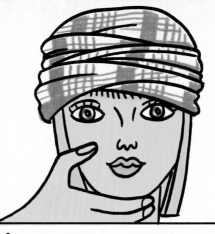

2. *Don't try to cover up*. Hair, like skin, reflects the state of your health. If you are lacking essential nutrients, if you are under stress or ill, your hair will show it.

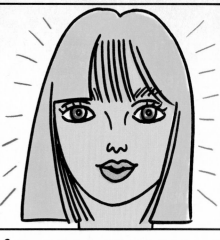

3. Because hair is a universal obsession and we all want that beautiful, healthy, shiny head of hair, we have a tendency to do too much to it or to do the wrong things.

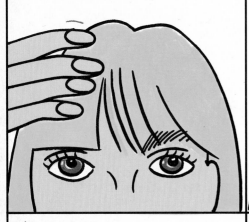

4. *Determining your hair type*. It's simple: if your skin is oily, probably your scalp is, too, since the scalp is an extension of your facial skin; and the condition of your scalp will determine the condition of your hair.

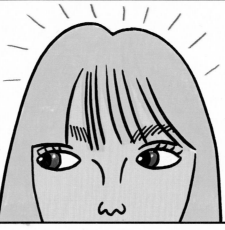

5. *Keep your scalp in good condition*. It's the best way to ensure healthy hair. If the pores in your scalp are clogged, the flow of oil is blocked, and you will get split ends, scalp infections, etc. To avoid this you must keep your scalp very clean.

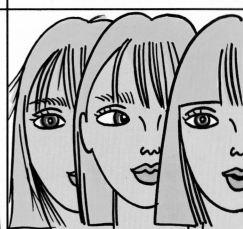

6. There are basically three types of hair: dry, normal, oily. Most people will fall under the dry or oily categories.

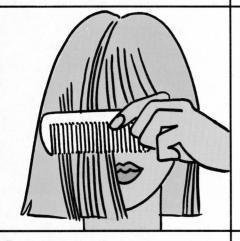

7. *Normal hair* should be bouncy, and have a sheen to it. It is definitely not oily, doesn't break easily when you brush or comb it, and is not overly elastic.

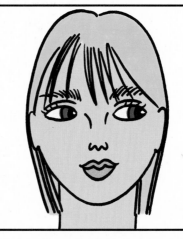

8. *Oily hair* looks oily, feels sleek, greasy, tends to stick together, looks limp, usually won't hold a set.

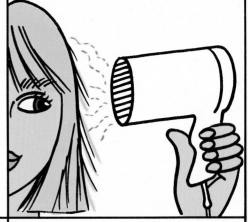

9. *Dry hair* lacks shine, elasticity, has a tendency to split, breaks easily, "frizzes." It doesn't retain water because the scalp is not functioning well. Dry hair can also result from damage caused by chemicals (coloring, overdone perm), or by the overuse of appliances.

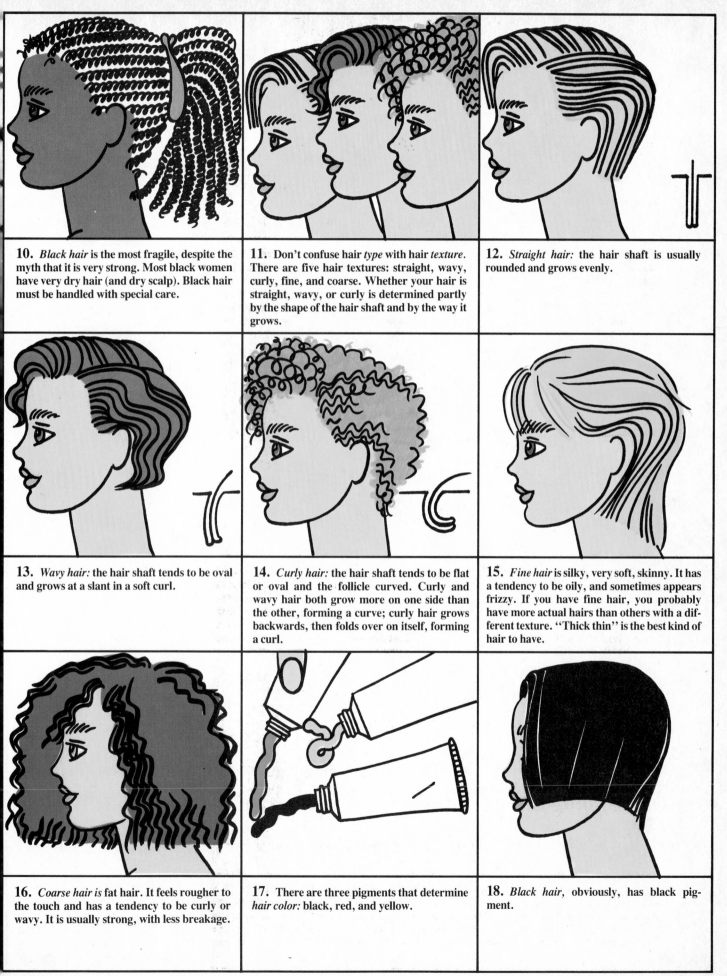

10. *Black hair* is the most fragile, despite the myth that it is very strong. Most black women have very dry hair (and dry scalp). Black hair must be handled with special care.

11. Don't confuse hair *type* with hair *texture*. There are five hair textures: straight, wavy, curly, fine, and coarse. Whether your hair is straight, wavy, or curly is determined partly by the shape of the hair shaft and by the way it grows.

12. *Straight hair:* the hair shaft is usually rounded and grows evenly.

13. *Wavy hair:* the hair shaft tends to be oval and grows at a slant in a soft curl.

14. *Curly hair:* the hair shaft tends to be flat or oval and the follicle curved. Curly and wavy hair both grow more on one side than the other, forming a curve; curly hair grows backwards, then folds over on itself, forming a curl.

15. *Fine hair* is silky, very soft, skinny. It has a tendency to be oily, and sometimes appears frizzy. If you have fine hair, you probably have more actual hairs than others with a different texture. "Thick thin" is the best kind of hair to have.

16. *Coarse hair is* fat hair. It feels rougher to the touch and has a tendency to be curly or wavy. It is usually strong, with less breakage.

17. There are three pigments that determine *hair color:* black, red, and yellow.

18. *Black hair,* obviously, has black pigment.

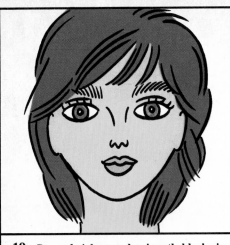

19. *Brown hair* has predominantly black pigment with strong traces of red or yellow.

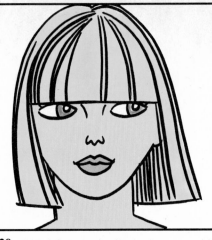

20. *Blond hair* has yellow pigment, with traces of red.

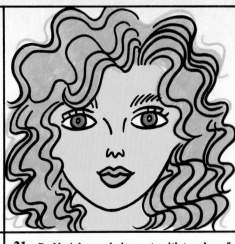

21. *Red hair* has red pigment, with touches of red and black.

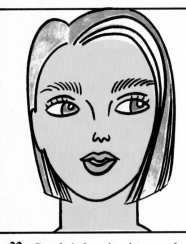

22. *Gray hair* doesn't exist as a color. It represents a loss of pigment.

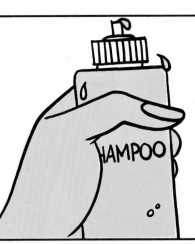

23. *How often should you shampoo?* It's the most important step toward clean, healthy hair, and we say—as routinely as you wash your body (which we hope is every day!) If you use the right shampoo (see #50, 52, 53), frequent shampooing can only benefit your hair.

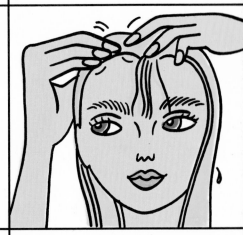

24. *The correct way to shampoo:* first wet your hair very thoroughly with warm water, massaging scalp gently with fingers for about 1 minute. This will prepare your scalp for the shampoo: it will unclog the pores, help the shampoo lather well, distribute it evenly.

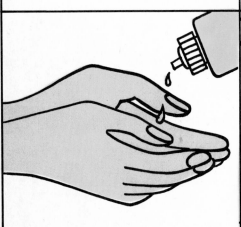

25. Pour a small amount of shampoo into the palm of your hand. Rub both hands together and apply to hair, concentrating primarily on the scalp area. (The scalp gets dirty faster than the hair.)

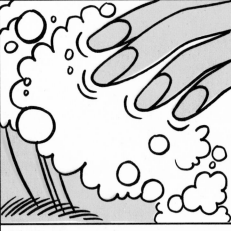

26. *Massage your scalp.* Use the tips of your fingers, never your nails. Move fingers over the entire scalp for about 5 minutes. This will also increase the circulation—very important for healthy hair.

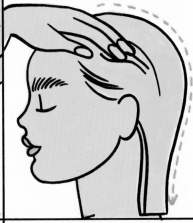

27. *Help to untangle hair* by running your fingers through your hair from scalp to ends. Alternate massaging and untangling movements.

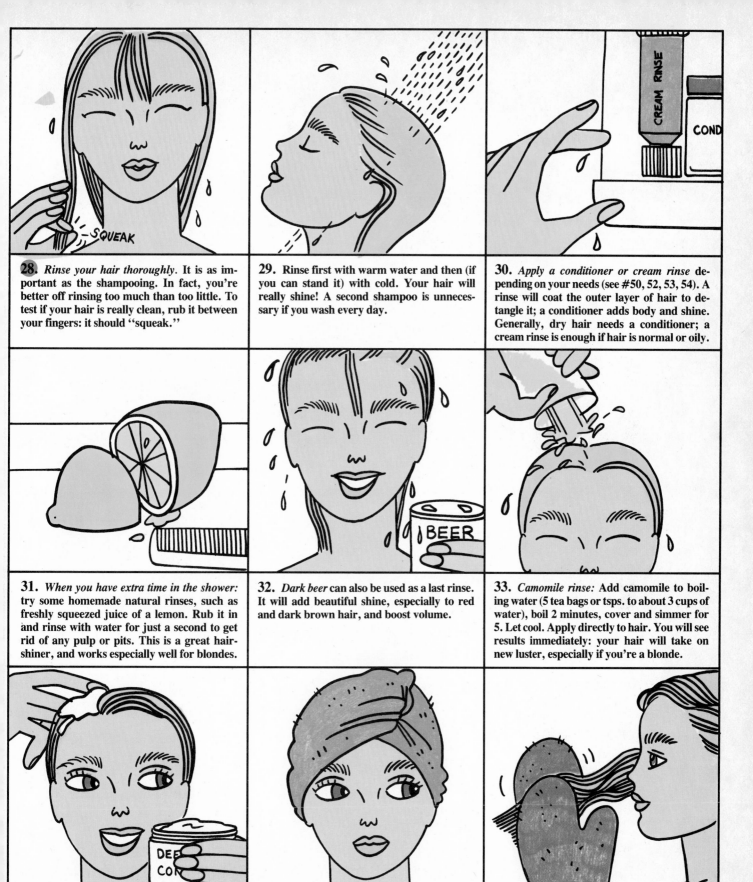

28. *Rinse your hair thoroughly.* It is as important as the shampooing. In fact, you're better off rinsing too much than too little. To test if your hair is really clean, rub it between your fingers: it should "squeak."

29. Rinse first with warm water and then (if you can stand it) with cold. Your hair will really shine! A second shampoo is unnecessary if you wash every day.

30. *Apply a conditioner or cream rinse* depending on your needs (see #50, 52, 53, 54). A rinse will coat the outer layer of hair to detangle it; a conditioner adds body and shine. Generally, dry hair needs a conditioner; a cream rinse is enough if hair is normal or oily.

31. *When you have extra time in the shower:* try some homemade natural rinses, such as freshly squeezed juice of a lemon. Rub it in and rinse with water for just a second to get rid of any pulp or pits. This is a great hair-shiner, and works especially well for blondes.

32. *Dark beer* can also be used as a last rinse. It will add beautiful shine, especially to red and dark brown hair, and boost volume.

33. *Camomile rinse:* Add camomile to boiling water (5 tea bags or tsps. to about 3 cups of water), boil 2 minutes, cover and simmer for 5. Let cool. Apply directly to hair. You will see results immediately: your hair will take on new luster, especially if you're a blonde.

34. *Deep-condition* when your hair is very dry or badly damaged by overuse of appliances, chemicals (coloring, perms), or by exposure to the environment. There is a variety of conditioners to choose from, from creams to oils. One will be right for you. (See also #55.)

35. *The correct way to dry:* You've probably never given this a thought, but do spend 2 minutes reading the following. First, pat dry with a clean towel and wrap towel around your head so it will absorb excess moisture. Be gentle; your hair is most vulnerable when wet.

36. *Try terry mittens.* You can buy them in your drugstore or department store; and use them instead of a towel to dry short hair, and for drying the ends of long hair.

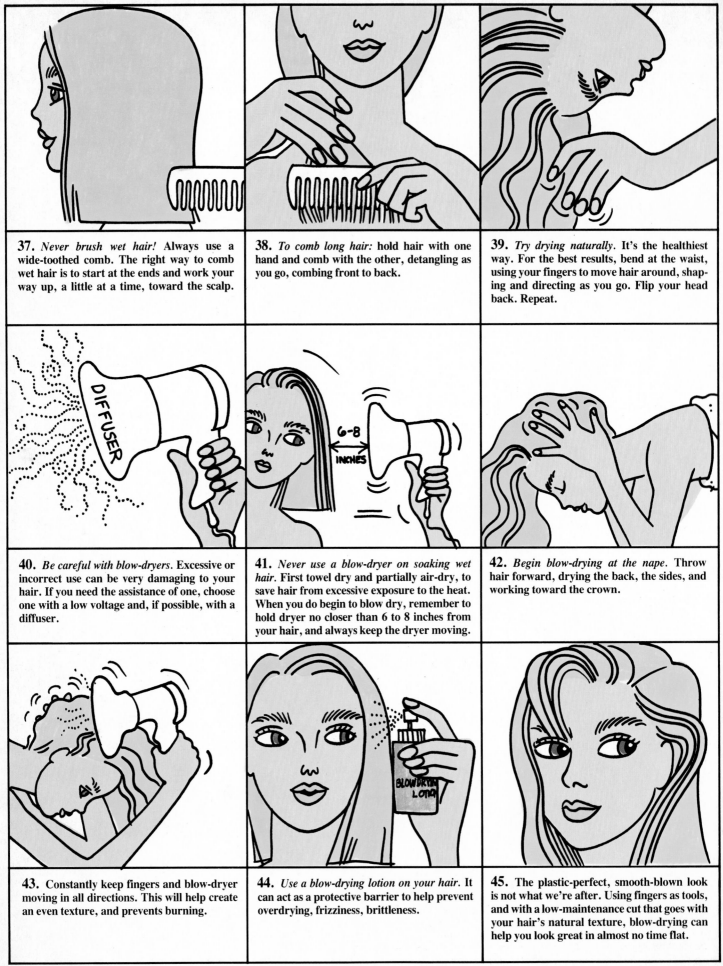

37. *Never brush wet hair!* Always use a wide-toothed comb. The right way to comb wet hair is to start at the ends and work your way up, a little at a time, toward the scalp.

38. *To comb long hair:* hold hair with one hand and comb with the other, detangling as you go, combing front to back.

39. *Try drying naturally.* It's the healthiest way. For the best results, bend at the waist, using your fingers to move hair around, shaping and directing as you go. Flip your head back. Repeat.

40. *Be careful with blow-dryers.* Excessive or incorrect use can be very damaging to your hair. If you need the assistance of one, choose one with a low voltage and, if possible, with a diffuser.

41. *Never use a blow-dryer on soaking wet hair.* First towel dry and partially air-dry, to save hair from excessive exposure to the heat. When you do begin to blow dry, remember to hold dryer no closer than 6 to 8 inches from your hair, and always keep the dryer moving.

42. *Begin blow-drying at the nape.* Throw hair forward, drying the back, the sides, and working toward the crown.

43. Constantly keep fingers and blow-dryer moving in all directions. This will help create an even texture, and prevents burning.

44. *Use a blow-drying lotion on your hair.* It can act as a protective barrier to help prevent overdrying, frizziness, brittleness.

45. The plastic-perfect, smooth-blown look is not what we're after. Using fingers as tools, and with a low-maintenance cut that goes with your hair's natural texture, blow-drying can help you look great in almost no time flat.

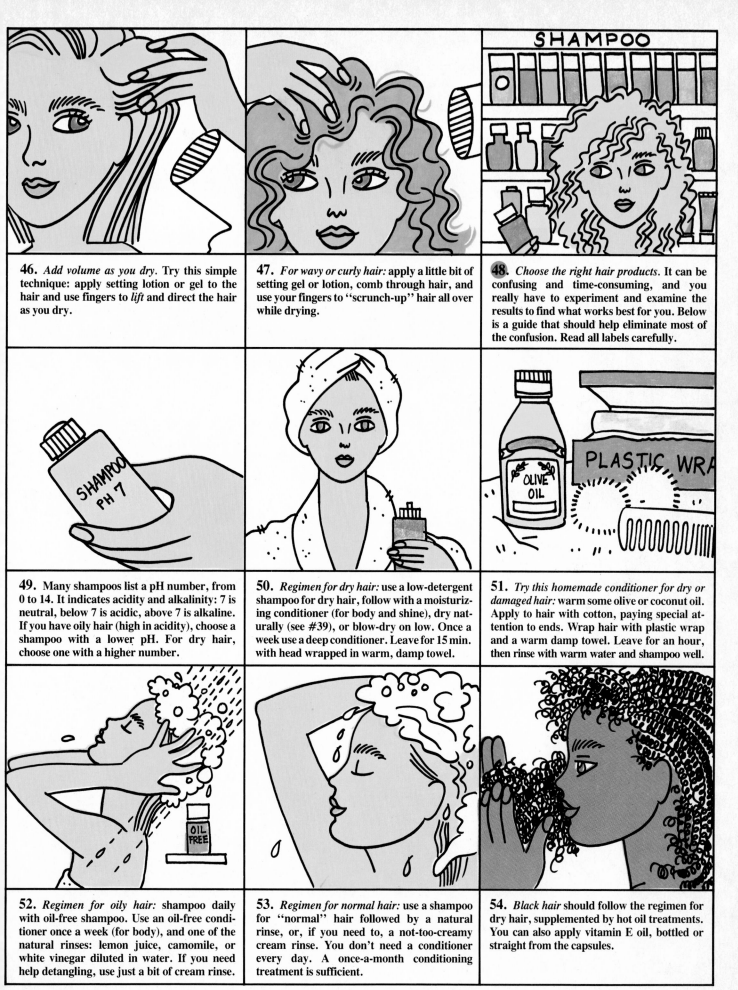

46. *Add volume as you dry.* Try this simple technique: apply setting lotion or gel to the hair and use fingers to *lift* and direct the hair as you dry.

47. *For wavy or curly hair:* apply a little bit of setting gel or lotion, comb through hair, and use your fingers to "scrunch-up" hair all over while drying.

48. *Choose the right hair products.* It can be confusing and time-consuming, and you really have to experiment and examine the results to find what works best for you. Below is a guide that should help eliminate most of the confusion. Read all labels carefully.

49. Many shampoos list a pH number, from 0 to 14. It indicates acidity and alkalinity: 7 is neutral, below 7 is acidic, above 7 is alkaline. If you have oily hair (high in acidity), choose a shampoo with a lower pH. For dry hair, choose one with a higher number.

50. *Regimen for dry hair:* use a low-detergent shampoo for dry hair, follow with a moisturizing conditioner (for body and shine), dry naturally (see #39), or blow-dry on low. Once a week use a deep conditioner. Leave for 15 min. with head wrapped in warm, damp towel.

51. *Try this homemade conditioner for dry or damaged hair:* warm some olive or coconut oil. Apply to hair with cotton, paying special attention to ends. Wrap hair with plastic wrap and a warm damp towel. Leave for an hour, then rinse with warm water and shampoo well.

52. *Regimen for oily hair:* shampoo daily with oil-free shampoo. Use an oil-free conditioner once a week (for body), and one of the natural rinses: lemon juice, camomile, or white vinegar diluted in water. If you need help detangling, use just a bit of cream rinse.

53. *Regimen for normal hair:* use a shampoo for "normal" hair followed by a natural rinse, or, if you need to, a not-too-creamy cream rinse. You don't need a conditioner every day. A once-a-month conditioning treatment is sufficient.

54. *Black hair* should follow the regimen for dry hair, supplemented by hot oil treatments. You can also apply vitamin E oil, bottled or straight from the capsules.

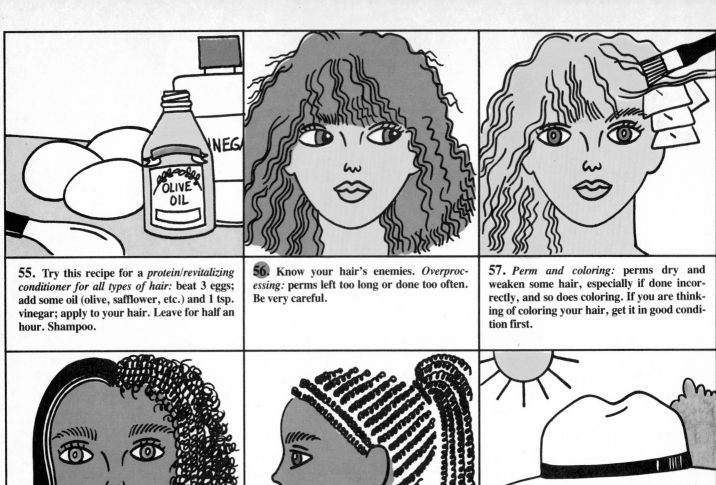

55. Try this recipe for a *protein/revitalizing conditioner for all types of hair:* beat 3 eggs; add some oil (olive, safflower, etc.) and 1 tsp. vinegar; apply to your hair. Leave for half an hour. Shampoo.

56. Know your hair's enemies. *Overprocessing:* perms left too long or done too often. Be very careful.

57. *Perm and coloring:* perms dry and weaken some hair, especially if done incorrectly, and so does coloring. If you are thinking of coloring your hair, get it in good condition first.

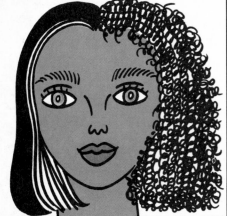

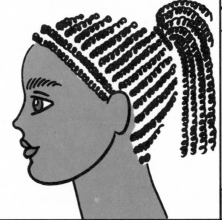

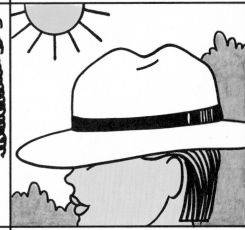

58. *Hair relaxers:* very damaging! If you have to use one, use a hair protector first. We think natural black hair is beautiful, and don't advise using anything to change the texture.

59. *Corn-rowing/tight ponytails:* excessive use can cause breakage and baldness, especially if they are continued for a long time.

60. *Sun exposure:* not only can sun burn the scalp, but it can dry out the hair and cause brittleness. It is especially damaging to color-treated hair and may change the color completely. Protect your hair with a hat or slick your hair back with deep conditioner.

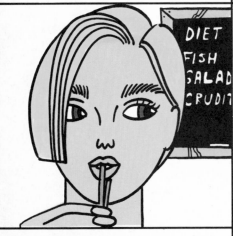

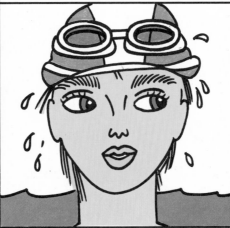

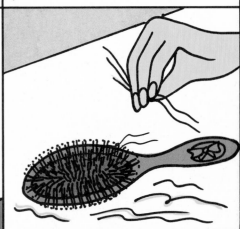

61. *A poor diet or chronic dieting:* may cause protein deficiency, which causes hair weakening and, in extreme cases, hair loss.

62. *Chlorine:* bleaches hair, dries out the ends, and may cause "split ends." It's a good idea to use a swim cap, or rinse hair with fresh water immediately after leaving the pool.

63. *Hair loss:* it's normal to lose 20 to 60 hairs a day. If you're losing more, you may have a problem (a deficiency in nutrients, or hormonal changes due to pregnancy, birth control pills, etc.). Excessive hair loss should be diagnosed by a dermatologist or trichologist.

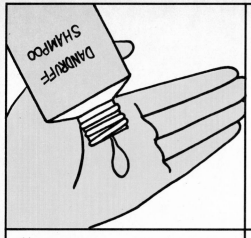

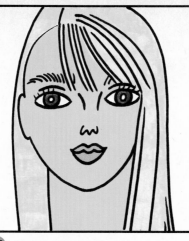

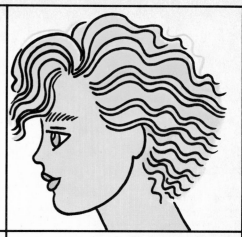

64. *Dandruff* is a condition in which the scalp sheds more than its normal share of dead skin cells. This can be caused by improper rinsing, overconditioning, sunburned scalp, or reactions to certain products. Good shampoos are available for this problem.

65. *The #1 rule of hair coloring:* stay in your natural color range. An extreme change, such as brown to light blond or vice versa, will look artificial and disrupt the balance of hair color and skin tone. Too much contrast between hair color and skin color can be aging.

66. We think of hair coloring the same way we think about make-up: it should enhance what's already there, not change it.

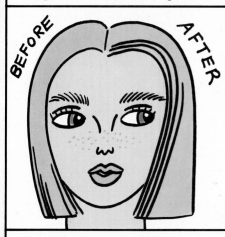

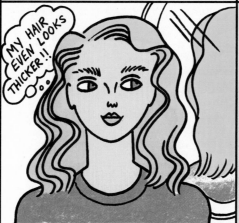

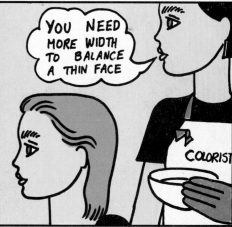

67. *Some unexpected benefits:* in certain instances, coloring can actually add body to your hair, especially if hair is fine or limp. Permanent coloring, for example, opens the cuticle, and as the color penetrates it swells the hair cortex. This gives hair the extra body.

68. Coloring can also make the hair look thicker and help get rid of excess oil. Henna does this: it coats the hair strands, adding thickness and shine.

69. A good colorist will know where to put warmer or darker tones to create the illusion of more volume where it's needed. Darker or warmer strands of hair can *look* fuller, and lighter strands can brighten up your face.

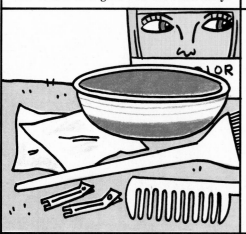

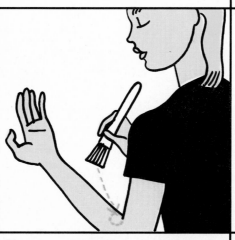

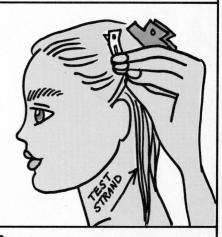

70. There are three types of hair-coloring techniques: permanent, semipermanent, and temporary. Before you or your colorist attempt any hair color, a skin patch test is a must to prevent possible allergic reactions.

71. *Skin patch test:* Dab some color on your skin; leave for 24 hours. If you notice any redness or skin irritation, it is an allergic reaction and under no circumstances should you use this product.

72. *At-home color test:* treat a small section of hair behind each ear. This will give you practice in applying the color properly, and you will be able to see if you like the way the color looks on you.

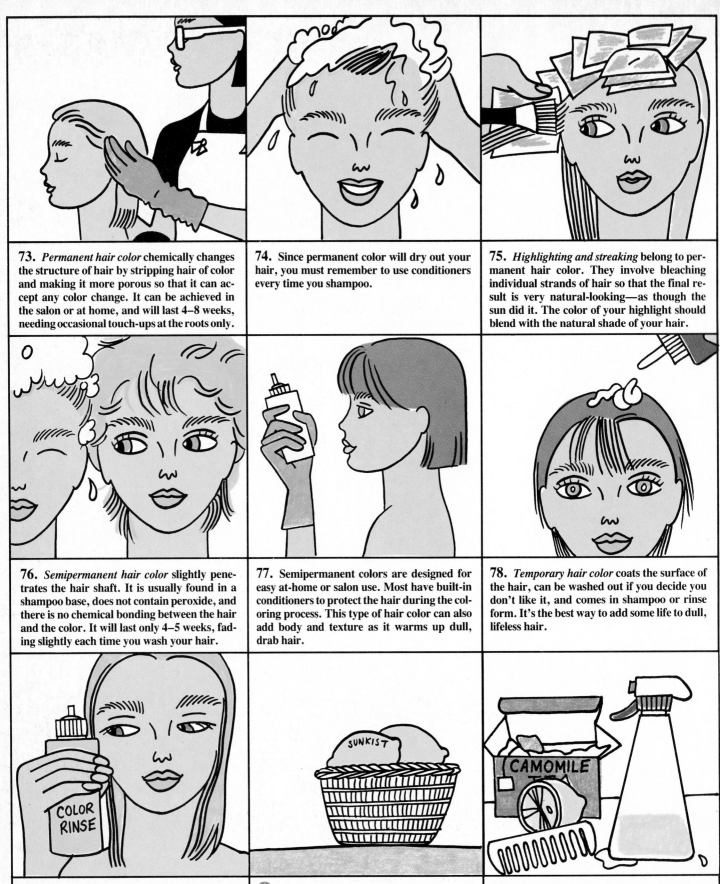

73. *Permanent hair color* chemically changes the structure of hair by stripping hair of color and making it more porous so that it can accept any color change. It can be achieved in the salon or at home, and will last 4–8 weeks, needing occasional touch-ups at the roots only.

74. Since permanent color will dry out your hair, you must remember to use conditioners every time you shampoo.

75. *Highlighting and streaking* belong to permanent hair color. They involve bleaching individual strands of hair so that the final result is very natural-looking—as though the sun did it. The color of your highlight should blend with the natural shade of your hair.

76. *Semipermanent hair color* slightly penetrates the hair shaft. It is usually found in a shampoo base, does not contain peroxide, and there is no chemical bonding between the hair and the color. It will last only 4–5 weeks, fading slightly each time you wash your hair.

77. Semipermanent colors are designed for easy at-home or salon use. Most have built-in conditioners to protect the hair during the coloring process. This type of hair color can also add body and texture as it warms up dull, drab hair.

78. *Temporary hair color* coats the surface of the hair, can be washed out if you decide you don't like it, and comes in shampoo or rinse form. It's the best way to add some life to dull, lifeless hair.

79. *Color rinse* is a temporary hair color, a water-soluble solution containing the weakest form of a hair dye. Applied immediately after shampooing, it can add a glow to your natural color and shampoos out easily.

80. *Natural hair enhancers:* there are several ways to give your hair a color "lift" without going through a chemical process and the expense involved. Here are our favorite recipes:

81. *For blondes:* dilute freshly squeezed lemon juice with water in a spray atomizer; spritz on hair for 10 minutes *before* shampooing. After shampooing, rinse normally. *Or,* brew some camomile tea, let it cool while you shampoo, then rinse through hair.

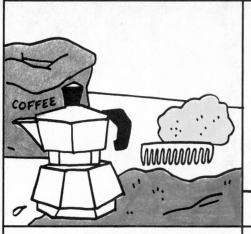

82. *For brunettes:* Brew espresso coffee. Cool. Rinse through hair before shampooing. After shampooing, follow up with a final cool water rinse, or rinse with diluted vinegar.

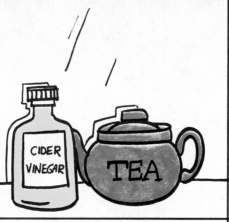

83. *For redheads:* Brew strong tea, cool, and rinse through hair to bring out highlights. *Or,* make a vinegar rinse using 6 parts water to 1 part cider vinegar.

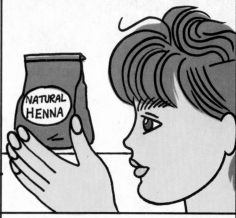

84. *Henna* (red, black, and neutral) is a permanent vegetable dye that coats hair without penetrating. Apply *only* to nonchemically colored hair. It will thicken hair and add shine! You can achieve excellent results at home, but the first application should be in a salon.

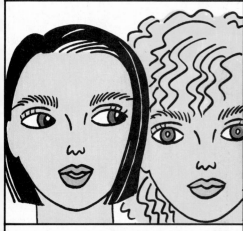

85. *If you are unhappy with your hair texture,* you can change it. There are basically two permanent techniques, permanents and hair straighteners, as well as many temporary ones (see #90, 97, 98, 102, 103, 105, 106, and ch. 4).

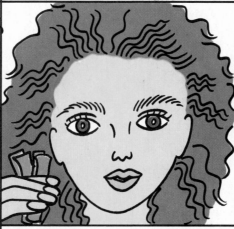

86. *A permanent* chemically alters the degree of curl in hair. It adds volume, frees you from time-consuming hair routines and gives you "wash-and-dry" hair. But your hair will require more pampering than usual, since permed hair can be extremely dry and breaks easily.

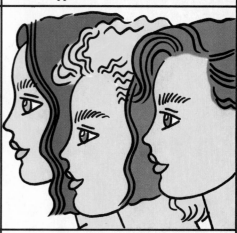

87. Think carefully about the look you want before perming, since any degree of curl is possible, from soft waves to tight curls.

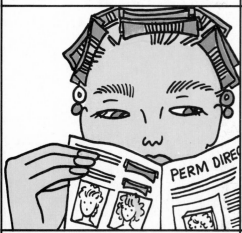

88. You can perm at home or in the salon. There are many "easy-to-use" perm products available. The rule is: read *all* labels and directions; don't leave the solution on a second more than indicated. Choose a time of day when you will not be interrupted.

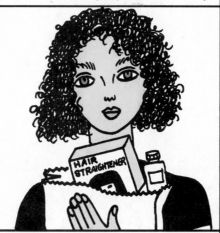

89. *Hair straightening* is the reverse chemical process of perming. A chemical solution is applied very close to the scalp so the hair appears straight. This process is dangerous and can cause hair loss.

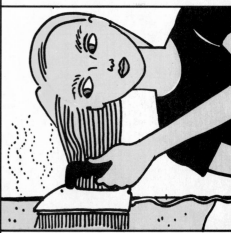

90. *Ironing:* You may laugh, but ironing really is the best way to get silky straight hair. Be sure to use the lowest temperature setting and don't iron too close to the scalp. Concentrate more at the ends. Remember, this is only for those with long hair!

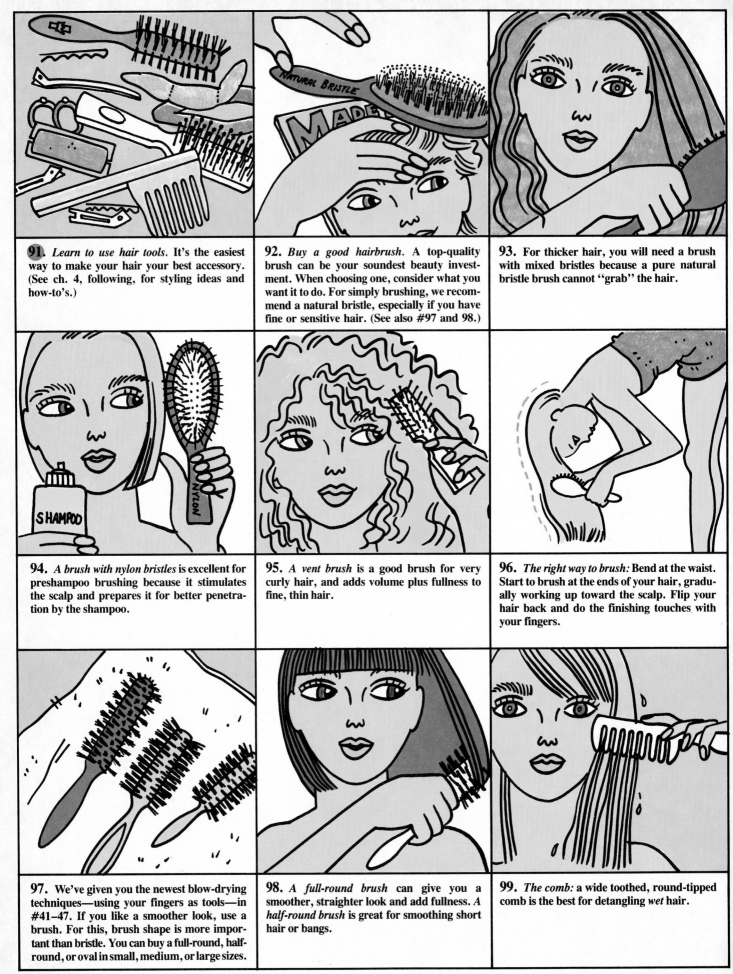

91. *Learn to use hair tools.* It's the easiest way to make your hair your best accessory. (See ch. 4, following, for styling ideas and how-to's.)

92. *Buy a good hairbrush.* A top-quality brush can be your soundest beauty investment. When choosing one, consider what you want it to do. For simply brushing, we recommend a natural bristle, especially if you have fine or sensitive hair. (See also #97 and 98.)

93. For thicker hair, you will need a brush with mixed bristles because a pure natural bristle brush cannot "grab" the hair.

94. *A brush with nylon bristles* is excellent for preshampoo brushing because it stimulates the scalp and prepares it for better penetration by the shampoo.

95. *A vent brush* is a good brush for very curly hair, and adds volume plus fullness to fine, thin hair.

96. *The right way to brush:* Bend at the waist. Start to brush at the ends of your hair, gradually working up toward the scalp. Flip your hair back and do the finishing touches with your fingers.

97. We've given you the newest blow-drying techniques—using your fingers as tools—in #41–47. If you like a smoother look, use a brush. For this, brush shape is more important than bristle. You can buy a full-round, half-round, or oval in small, medium, or large sizes.

98. *A full-round brush* can give you a smoother, straighter look and add fullness. *A half-round brush* is great for smoothing short hair or bangs.

99. *The comb:* a wide toothed, round-tipped comb is the best for detangling *wet* hair.

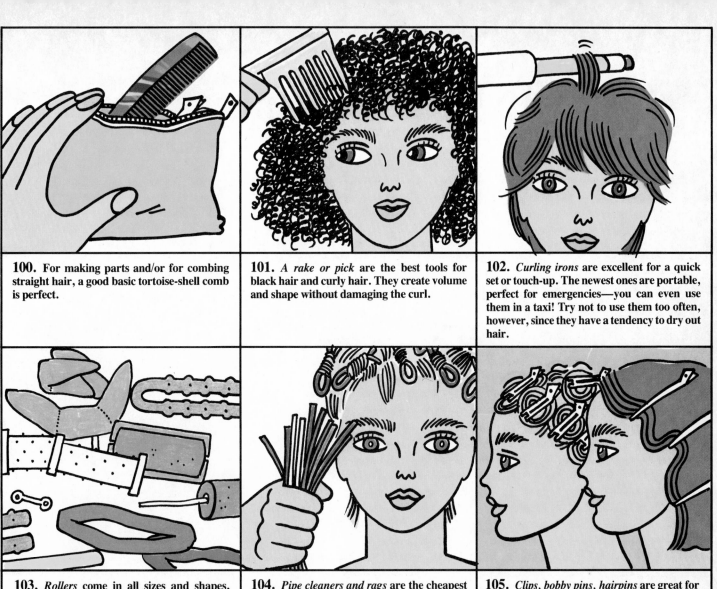

100. For making parts and/or for combing straight hair, a good basic tortoise-shell comb is perfect.

101. *A rake or pick* are the best tools for black hair and curly hair. They create volume and shape without damaging the curl.

102. *Curling irons* are excellent for a quick set or touch-up. The newest ones are portable, perfect for emergencies—you can even use them in a taxi! Try not to use them too often, however, since they have a tendency to dry out hair.

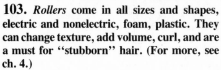

103. *Rollers* come in all sizes and shapes, electric and nonelectric, foam, plastic. They can change texture, add volume, curl, and are a must for "stubborn" hair. (For more, see ch. 4.)

104. *Pipe cleaners and rags* are the cheapest alternative to store-bought hair rollers. They're easy to use and nondamaging to hair. (For more, see ch. 4.)

105. *Clips, bobby pins, hairpins* are great for building in waves and curls. The less hair in each curl, the tighter the curl. (For more, see ch. 4.)

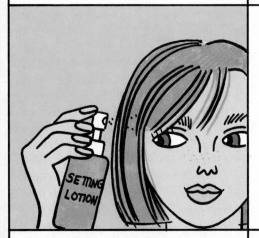

106. *Gels, setting lotions.* These are the newest hair products. Use them with your fingers to push hair into shape, control, add volume and direction. They are also excellent helpers for other hair tools, such as dryers, curlers, brushes. (See ch. 4 for more.)

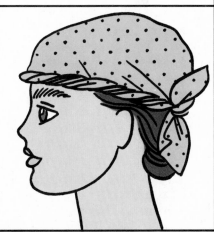

107. *Scarves, fabrics.* Use them to protect your hair from the elements, when you want your hair out of the way—or on days when it simply won't behave. Just pull out a scarf, and wrap. (See ch. 4 for various techniques.)

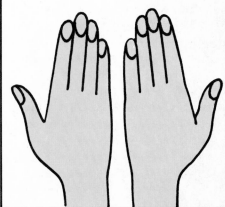

108. *Learn to use your hands.* They are the best hair tools you have. Use them with gels, sprays, setting lotions, rollers, blow-dryers—to mold, add volume, style, and for last minute touch-ups.

4
HAIR STYLING

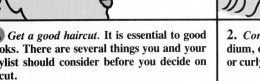

1. *Get a good haircut.* It is essential to good looks. There are several things you and your stylist should consider before you decide on a cut.

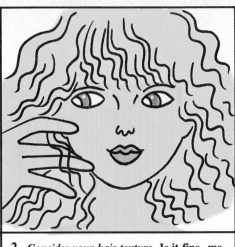

2. *Consider your hair texture.* Is it fine, medium, or coarse? Is your hair straight, wavy, or curly? (See p. 41, #11–16 for more.)

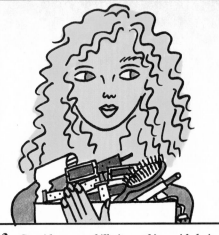

3. *Consider your skills in working with hair.* How adept are you with a blow-dryer, a curling iron, electric rollers? Do you want to work with hair tools—or do you just want "wash-and-dry" hair?

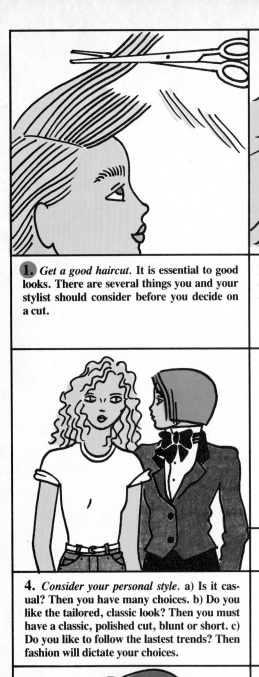

4. *Consider your personal style.* a) Is it casual? Then you have many choices. b) Do you like the tailored, classic look? Then you must have a classic, polished cut, blunt or short. c) Do you like to follow the lastest trends? Then fashion will dictate your choices.

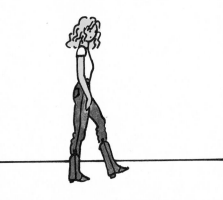

5. *Consider your body proportions.* If you are short, you shouldn't have very long, voluminous hair. If you are overweight, or generally round, a short cut may not be the best for you.

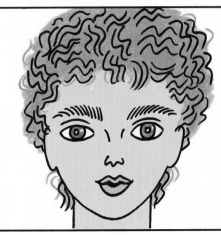

6. Haircuts fall into three general categories. The *short cut* ends anywhere from the tip of the ears to the chin. Getting a short cut is a big decision, but the effect can be stunning. The short cut opens up your face and can reveal qualities you never knew existed.

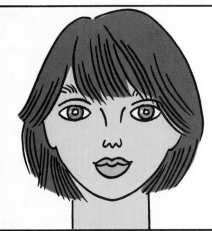

7. The *medium cut* is hair that falls anywhere from the chin to the shoulders. It is truly the "happy medium"—the safest choice if you don't want long hair but are afraid of the short cut.

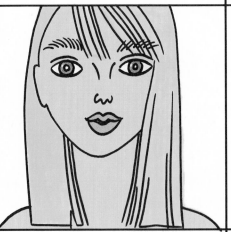

8. The *long cut* is shoulder-length or longer.

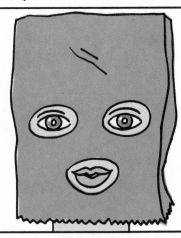

9. *Are you unhappy with your cut?* There is no need to go around with your head in a paper bag. Remember—a cut is not forever. Your hair will grow out, and until it does there are many things you can do to make it look good. Just keep reading . . .

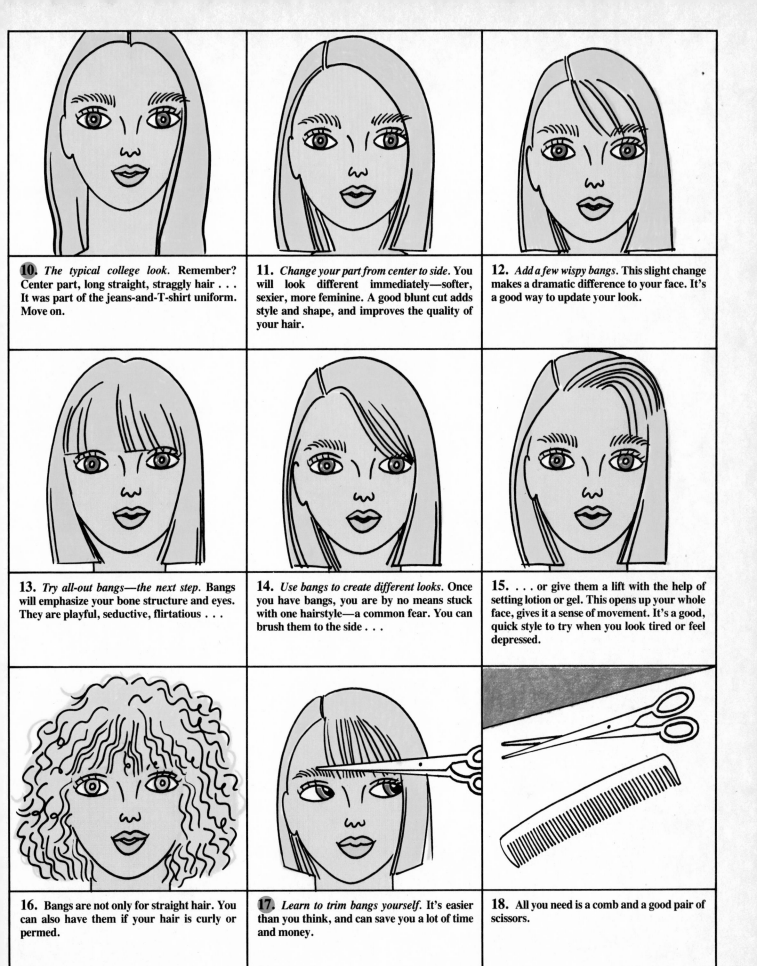

10. *The typical college look.* Remember? Center part, long straight, straggly hair . . . It was part of the jeans-and-T-shirt uniform. Move on.

11. *Change your part from center to side.* You will look different immediately—softer, sexier, more feminine. A good blunt cut adds style and shape, and improves the quality of your hair.

12. *Add a few wispy bangs.* This slight change makes a dramatic difference to your face. It's a good way to update your look.

13. *Try all-out bangs—the next step.* Bangs will emphasize your bone structure and eyes. They are playful, seductive, flirtatious . . .

14. *Use bangs to create different looks.* Once you have bangs, you are by no means stuck with one hairstyle—a common fear. You can brush them to the side . . .

15. . . . or give them a lift with the help of setting lotion or gel. This opens up your whole face, gives it a sense of movement. It's a good, quick style to try when you look tired or feel depressed.

16. Bangs are not only for straight hair. You can also have them if your hair is curly or permed.

17. *Learn to trim bangs yourself.* It's easier than you think, and can save you a lot of time and money.

18. All you need is a comb and a good pair of scissors.

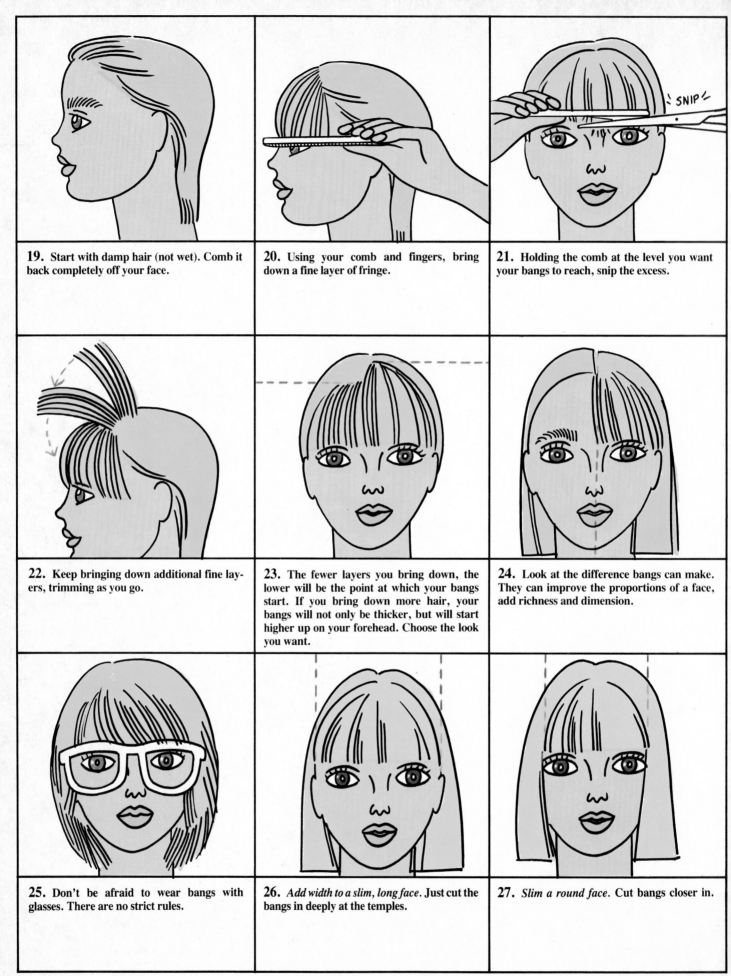

19. Start with damp hair (not wet). Comb it back completely off your face.

20. Using your comb and fingers, bring down a fine layer of fringe.

21. Holding the comb at the level you want your bangs to reach, snip the excess.

SNIP

22. Keep bringing down additional fine layers, trimming as you go.

23. The fewer layers you bring down, the lower will be the point at which your bangs start. If you bring down more hair, your bangs will not only be thicker, but will start higher up on your forehead. Choose the look you want.

24. Look at the difference bangs can make. They can improve the proportions of a face, add richness and dimension.

25. Don't be afraid to wear bangs with glasses. There are no strict rules.

26. *Add width to a slim, long face.* Just cut the bangs in deeply at the temples.

27. *Slim a round face.* Cut bangs closer in.

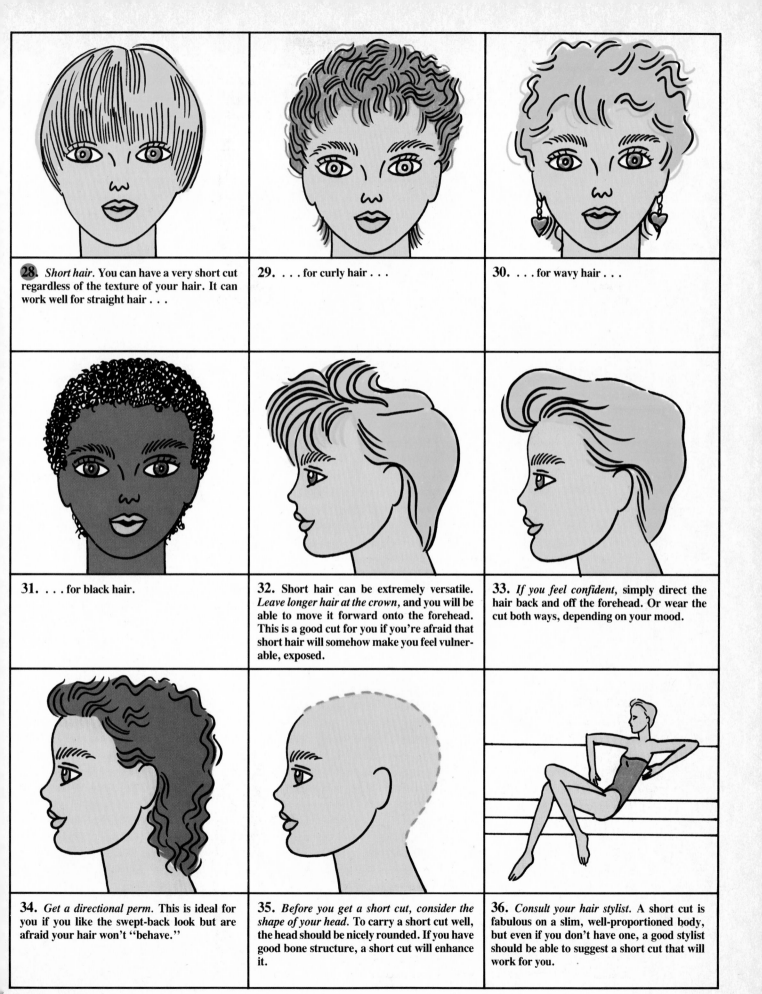

28. *Short hair.* You can have a very short cut regardless of the texture of your hair. It can work well for straight hair . . .

29. . . . for curly hair . . .

30. . . . for wavy hair . . .

31. . . . for black hair.

32. Short hair can be extremely versatile. *Leave longer hair at the crown,* and you will be able to move it forward onto the forehead. This is a good cut for you if you're afraid that short hair will somehow make you feel vulnerable, exposed.

33. *If you feel confident,* simply direct the hair back and off the forehead. Or wear the cut both ways, depending on your mood.

34. *Get a directional perm.* This is ideal for you if you like the swept-back look but are afraid your hair won't "behave."

35. *Before you get a short cut, consider the shape of your head.* To carry a short cut well, the head should be nicely rounded. If you have good bone structure, a short cut will enhance it.

36. *Consult your hair stylist.* A short cut is fabulous on a slim, well-proportioned body, but even if you don't have one, a good stylist should be able to suggest a short cut that will work for you.

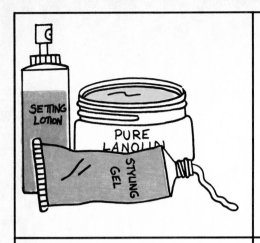

37. *Invest in setting lotion, gel, and pure lanolin.* They will help you get the most out of your short hair.

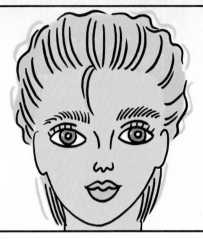

38. *Move hair away from the face.* If you like this look, here is a simple method: put a dab of pure lanolin on your hand, rub hands together . . .

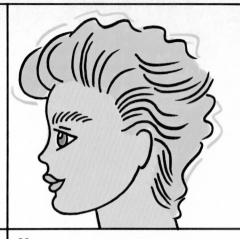

39. . . . and comb hands backward through the hair. The results are dramatic. Your hair will have great sheen and style—especially fitting for a glamorous evening.

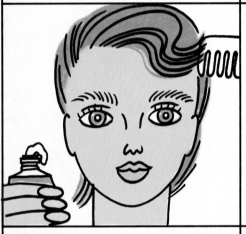

40. *Create a front wave.* Comb some setting gel into damp hair, push hair into the shape you want . . .

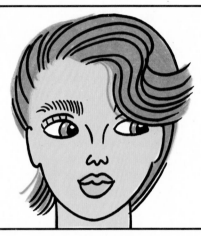

41. . . . and when you achieve the desired curve, finish drying hair (naturally or with a blow-dryer set on gentle), then comb through lightly.

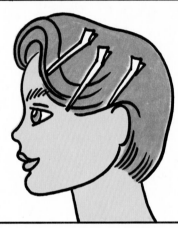

42. *For more waves:* use the technique in #40 and 41, but add long clips as you shape the hair. Remove when hair is dry.

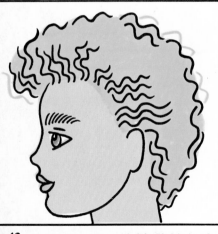

43. *No-maintenance with lift.* If this is what you want, a permanent is the key.

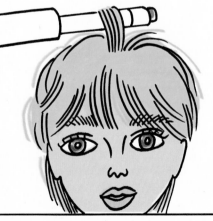

44. *Use a curling iron.* It's an easy way to give your hair a quick temporary lift. (See p. 51 , #102 for more.)

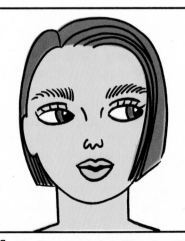

45. *For fine, straight hair.* If you have it, this classic short blunt cut is best for you. With only minimal maintenance, your hair will always look polished and sleek.

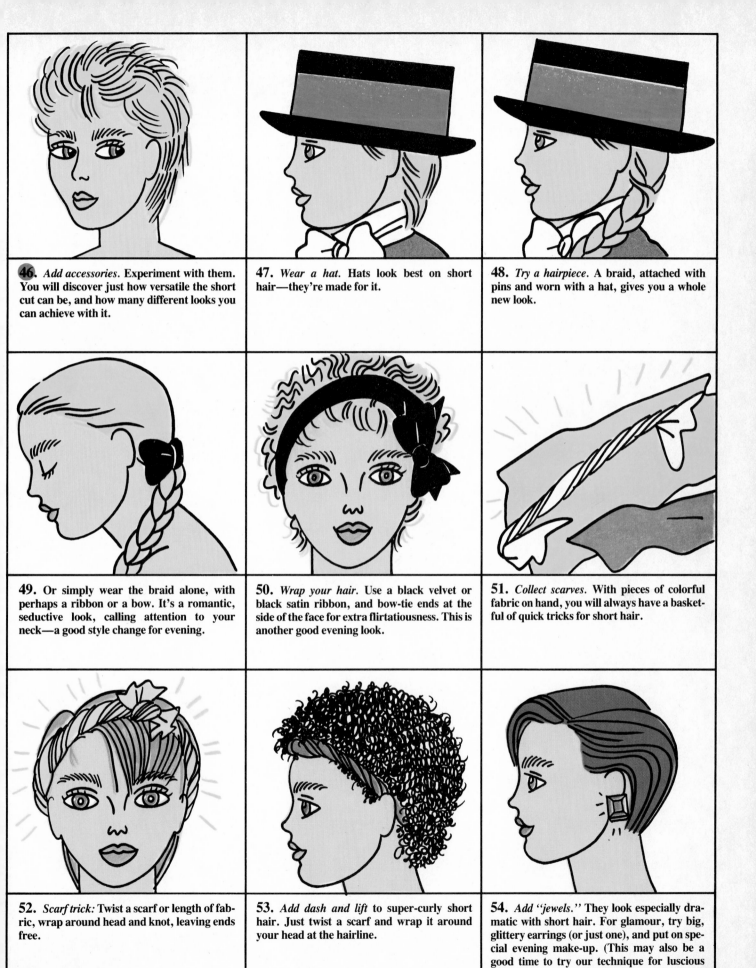

46. *Add accessories*. Experiment with them. You will discover just how versatile the short cut can be, and how many different looks you can achieve with it.

47. *Wear a hat*. Hats look best on short hair—they're made for it.

48. *Try a hairpiece*. A braid, attached with pins and worn with a hat, gives you a whole new look.

49. Or simply wear the braid alone, with perhaps a ribbon or a bow. It's a romantic, seductive look, calling attention to your neck—a good style change for evening.

50. *Wrap your hair*. Use a black velvet or black satin ribbon, and bow-tie ends at the side of the face for extra flirtatiousness. This is another good evening look.

51. *Collect scarves*. With pieces of colorful fabric on hand, you will always have a basketful of quick tricks for short hair.

52. *Scarf trick:* Twist a scarf or length of fabric, wrap around head and knot, leaving ends free.

53. *Add dash and lift* to super-curly short hair. Just twist a scarf and wrap it around your head at the hairline.

54. *Add "jewels."* They look especially dramatic with short hair. For glamour, try big, glittery earrings (or just one), and put on special evening make-up. (This may also be a good time to try our technique for luscious lips; see p. 35 , #136–138).

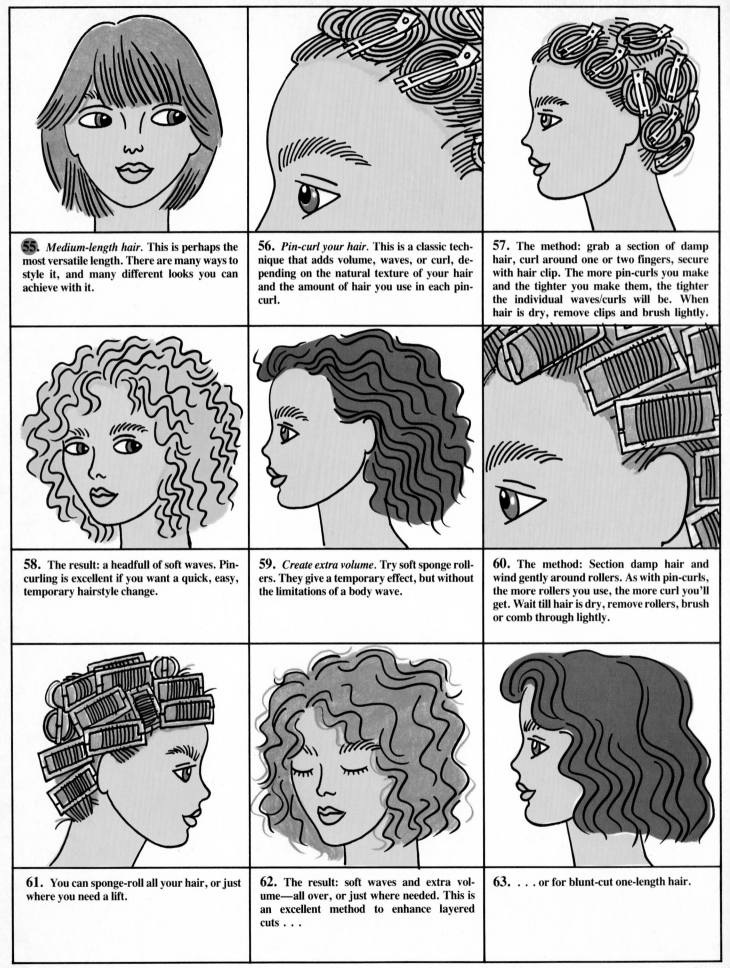

55. *Medium-length hair.* This is perhaps the most versatile length. There are many ways to style it, and many different looks you can achieve with it.

56. *Pin-curl your hair.* This is a classic technique that adds volume, waves, or curl, depending on the natural texture of your hair and the amount of hair you use in each pin-curl.

57. The method: grab a section of damp hair, curl around one or two fingers, secure with hair clip. The more pin-curls you make and the tighter you make them, the tighter the individual waves/curls will be. When hair is dry, remove clips and brush lightly.

58. The result: a headfull of soft waves. Pin-curling is excellent if you want a quick, easy, temporary hairstyle change.

59. *Create extra volume.* Try soft sponge rollers. They give a temporary effect, but without the limitations of a body wave.

60. The method: Section damp hair and wind gently around rollers. As with pin-curls, the more rollers you use, the more curl you'll get. Wait till hair is dry, remove rollers, brush or comb through lightly.

61. You can sponge-roll all your hair, or just where you need a lift.

62. The result: soft waves and extra volume—all over, or just where needed. This is an excellent method to enhance layered cuts . . .

63. . . . or for blunt-cut one-length hair.

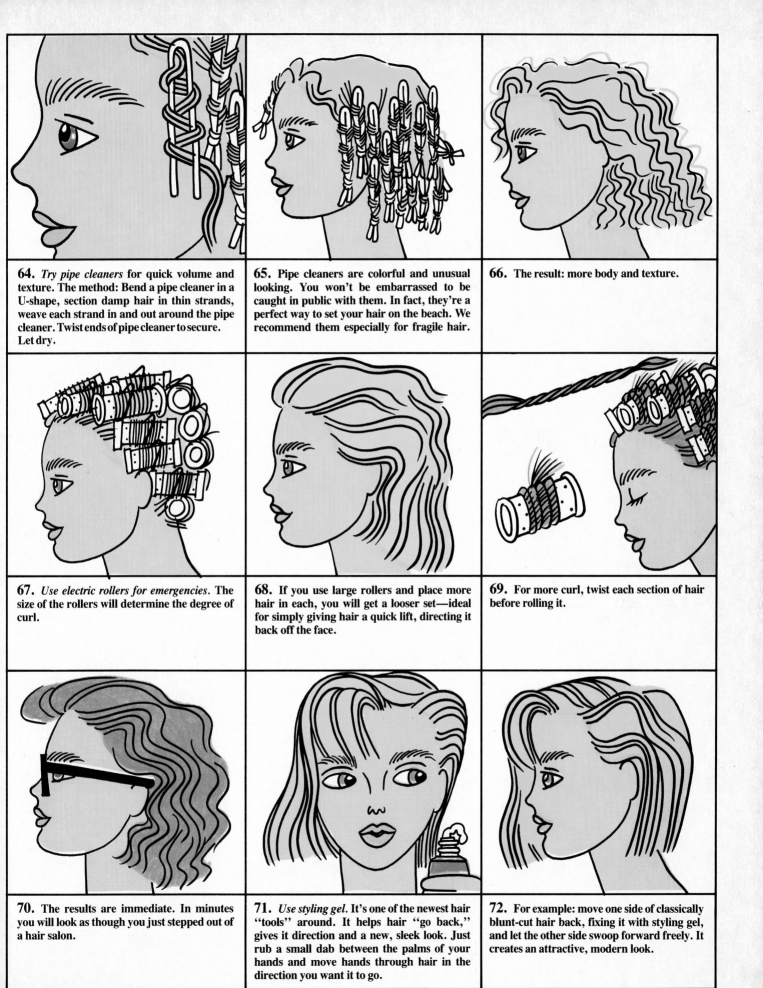

64. *Try pipe cleaners* for quick volume and texture. The method: Bend a pipe cleaner in a U-shape, section damp hair in thin strands, weave each strand in and out around the pipe cleaner. Twist ends of pipe cleaner to secure. Let dry.

65. Pipe cleaners are colorful and unusual looking. You won't be embarrassed to be caught in public with them. In fact, they're a perfect way to set your hair on the beach. We recommend them especially for fragile hair.

66. The result: more body and texture.

67. *Use electric rollers for emergencies.* The size of the rollers will determine the degree of curl.

68. If you use large rollers and place more hair in each, you will get a looser set—ideal for simply giving hair a quick lift, directing it back off the face.

69. For more curl, twist each section of hair before rolling it.

70. The results are immediate. In minutes you will look as though you just stepped out of a hair salon.

71. *Use styling gel.* It's one of the newest hair "tools" around. It helps hair "go back," gives it direction and a new, sleek look. Just rub a small dab between the palms of your hands and move hands through hair in the direction you want it to go.

72. For example: move one side of classically blunt-cut hair back, fixing it with styling gel, and let the other side swoop forward freely. It creates an attractive, modern look.

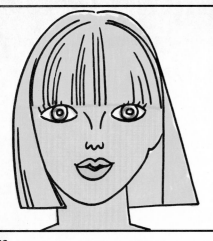

73. *Blunt cut with bangs.* This is a good choice for medium-length hair that is straight, shiny, and healthy.

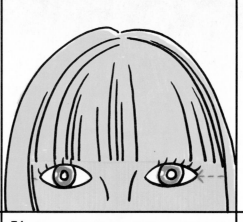

74. *Asymmetrical bangs.* Cut bangs 1″ deeper on one side *only*. This helps hair move, and adds something extra to a classic cut.

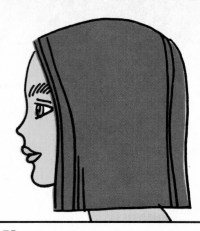

75. *Another medium-length classic:* perfectly blunt-cut, side-parted hair, all line and sleekness. You will achieve best results with this cut if your hair is straight.

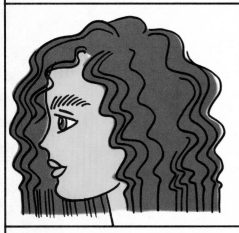

76. *The wavy blunt cut.* If you have enough natural texture, this can be an easy, minimal-maintenance style for you.

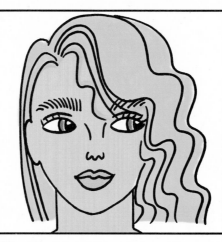

77. *Seductive asymmetry.* Side part the hair, tuck one side behind the ear, and leave soft waves cascading down on the other. This is a favorite with many men . . .

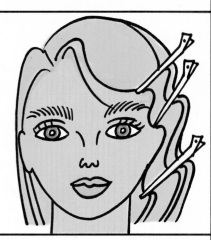

78. *Make waves,* or accentuate natural ones, by clipping damp hair with large clips.

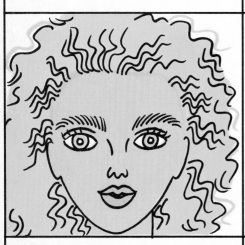

79. *A soft mane of waves.* Curly/coarse medium-length hair looks wonderful directed off the face, especially if you have good features.

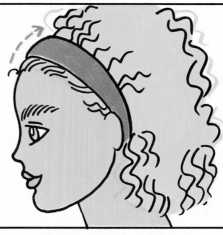

80. The method: apply a hint of setting lotion, direct hair back with a hairband, and blow-dry in place. Remove band, bend forward, brush gently, and flip hair back.

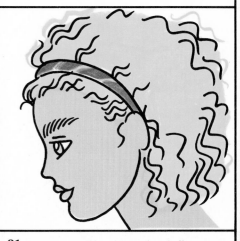

81. *A pretty hairband,* tortoise-shell or perhaps suede, can discreetly "set" hair all day long. For a splendid P.M. look, just remove band and brush hair lightly.

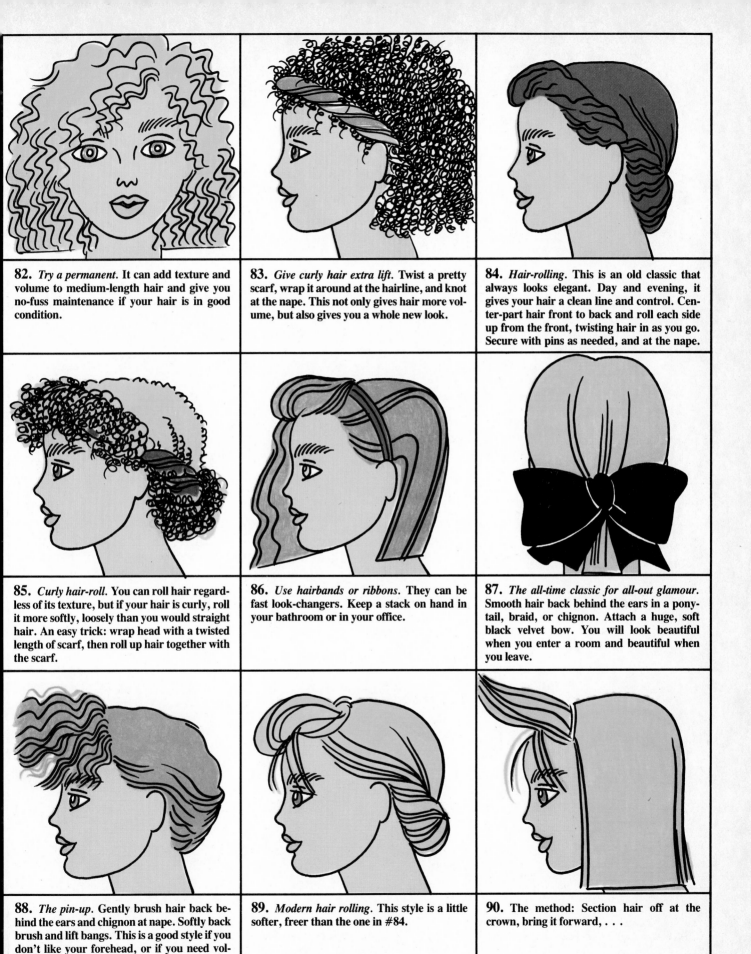

82. *Try a permanent.* It can add texture and volume to medium-length hair and give you no-fuss maintenance if your hair is in good condition.

83. *Give curly hair extra lift.* Twist a pretty scarf, wrap it around at the hairline, and knot at the nape. This not only gives hair more volume, but also gives you a whole new look.

84. *Hair-rolling.* This is an old classic that always looks elegant. Day and evening, it gives your hair a clean line and control. Center-part hair front to back and roll each side up from the front, twisting hair in as you go. Secure with pins as needed, and at the nape.

85. *Curly hair-roll.* You can roll hair regardless of its texture, but if your hair is curly, roll it more softly, loosely than you would straight hair. An easy trick: wrap head with a twisted length of scarf, then roll up hair together with the scarf.

86. *Use hairbands or ribbons.* They can be fast look-changers. Keep a stack on hand in your bathroom or in your office.

87. *The all-time classic for all-out glamour.* Smooth hair back behind the ears in a ponytail, braid, or chignon. Attach a huge, soft black velvet bow. You will look beautiful when you enter a room and beautiful when you leave.

88. *The pin-up.* Gently brush hair back behind the ears and chignon at nape. Softly back brush and lift bangs. This is a good style if you don't like your forehead, or if you need volume in the front.

89. *Modern hair rolling.* This style is a little softer, freer than the one in #84.

90. The method: Section hair off at the crown, bring it forward, . . .

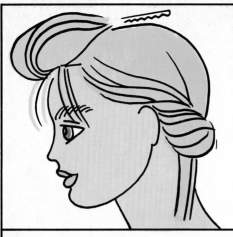

91. . . . and softly, loosely twist back and pin to secure. Center-part remainder of hair and roll up and back, twisting hair in as you go.

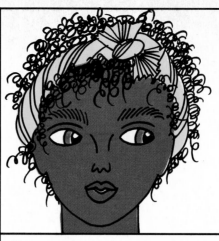

92. *Wrap curly hair.* Just twist a length of fabric or a scarf or two together, encircling head at hairline.

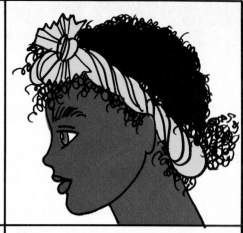

93. Then knot hair at the nape, make a chignon, or pin hair inside the twisted fabric. This can be especially beautiful for evening. Try it with glittery scarves, silk, or combine fabrics and textures.

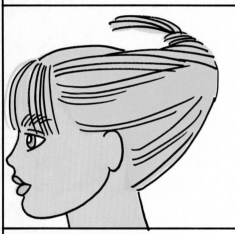

94. *A quick change for evening.* Smooth all hair back, twist up loosely, . . .

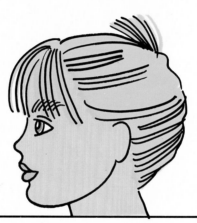

95. . . . and pin to secure at crown, leaving ends free.

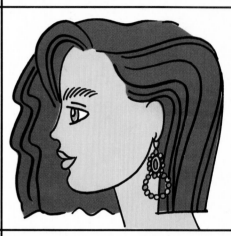

96. *Evening glamour.* On damp hair, use a spritz of setting lotion to direct hair back and off the face behind one ear. Let dry, then gently brush through. Add a "stopper" of an earring.

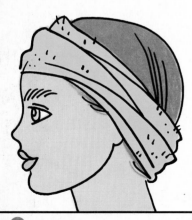

97. *For sport or play:* smooth all hair back (you can "help" it with setting lotion or gel) and wrap head with a soft fabric or scarf (you can even use a cut-up old T-shirt, a strip of bed sheet or towel). This is also a good after-shampoo look, while hair is damp.

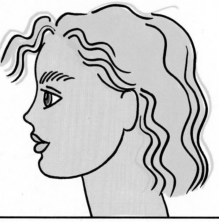

98. A variation that also works for day, evening or beach: first, bring a few short wisps of hair forward, . . .

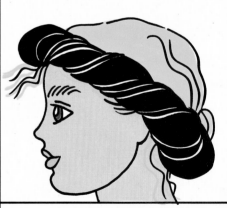

99. . . . then twist the fabric or scarf and wrap head as in #97.

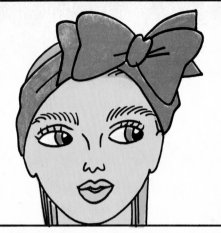

100. *An attention-getter.* Take a long swatch of soft fabric or a chiffon scarf or two, wrap head, and end in a huge bow.

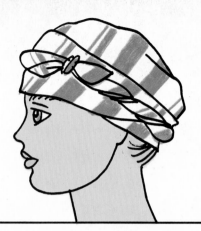

101. *When you hate your hair.* Wrap head completely with an oversize scarf. Fold it in a triangle, placing center of fold low on forehead (thin cotton or gauze work particularly well). Bring two sides back, shaping scarf to head as you go. Twist ends, and knot in front.

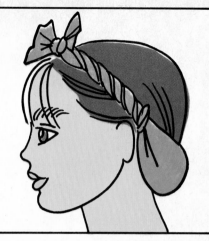

102. *Make a pocket.* This works well for the beach if you use a lightweight cotton or gauze. Switch to a shimmery fabric, and the look can go evening.

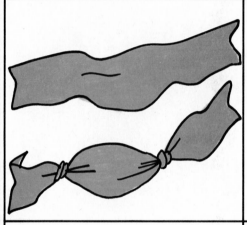

103. The method: take a long scarf in a flexible lightweight fabric and knot twice to form a center pocket.

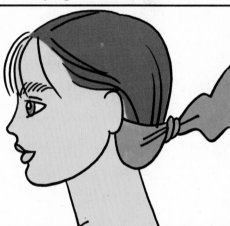

104. Smooth hair back behind the ears, tuck ends into the scarf-pocket, . . .

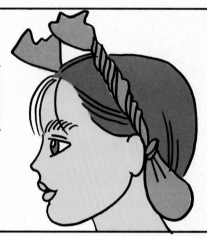

105. . . . and twist up ends of scarf, tying them at the crown.

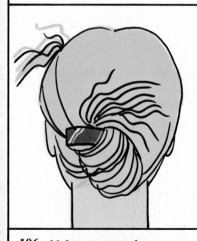

106. *Make an everyday gesture special.* Everyone with medium to long hair sometimes wants to lift it up and off the neck: hair is smoothed back off the ears and barretted in place. Instead, smooth hair back, grab the "tail" and loosely give it one twist . . .

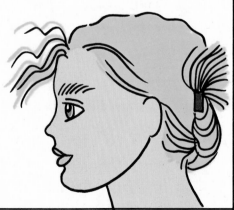

107. Barrette in place leaving ends free. You can use a classic tortoise shell barrette or go for something eye-catching—enameled, sequined.

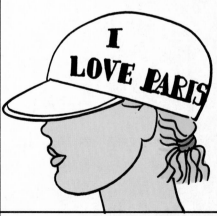

108. *A different look for beach/sport/play.* Pull all hair back in a "tail," braid, or baby chignon, and pull on a funny cap or hat.

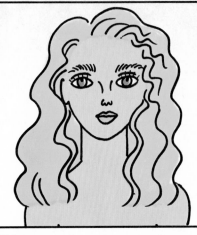

109. *Long hair*. You should have it only if your hair is beautiful and in good condition. And remember: even if you want to keep your hair long, an occasional trim is a must.

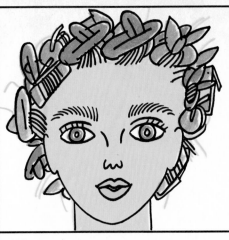

110. *Try soft rollers*. They come in every shape and color, and give long hair volume and wave, gently, without damaging it. Use on damp hair. You can sleep in soft rollers, and some are even pretty enough for a beach-set.

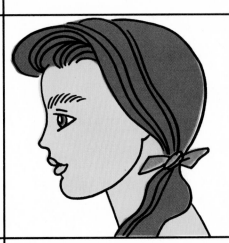

111. When you remove them, you'll have soft, ripply waves of hair.

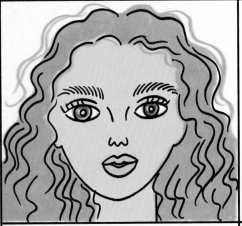

112. *Give thick long hair extra "oomph" with the braid-set*—or use this when you don't want to be bothered with any hair tools.

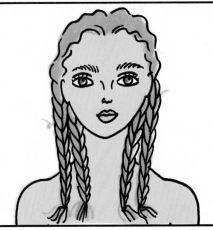

113. The method: simply braid damp hair, let dry. The fewer and the fatter the braids, the looser the wave you'll get. You can do two braids, four, eight . . . Do it in the evening for an overnight set, or use the braids as a daytime hairdo and un-do for evening waves.

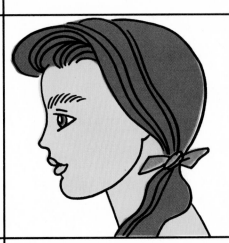

114. *Instant polish*. Softly pull hair back and catch at nape with a soft ribbon, a touch of suede, leather, or lace.

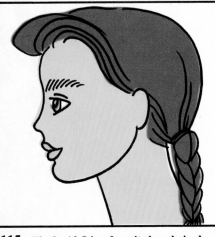

115. *The braid*. It's a favorite long hair classic. Pull hair back, divide into three sections and braid.

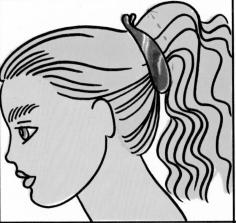

116. *The ponytail*. Try it with a long barrette. Used vertically it creates an entirely new silhouette and gives the illusion of greater hair volume.

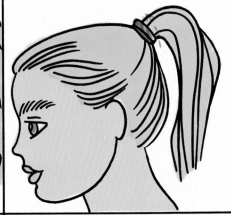

117. *The standard ponytail*. Notice the difference?

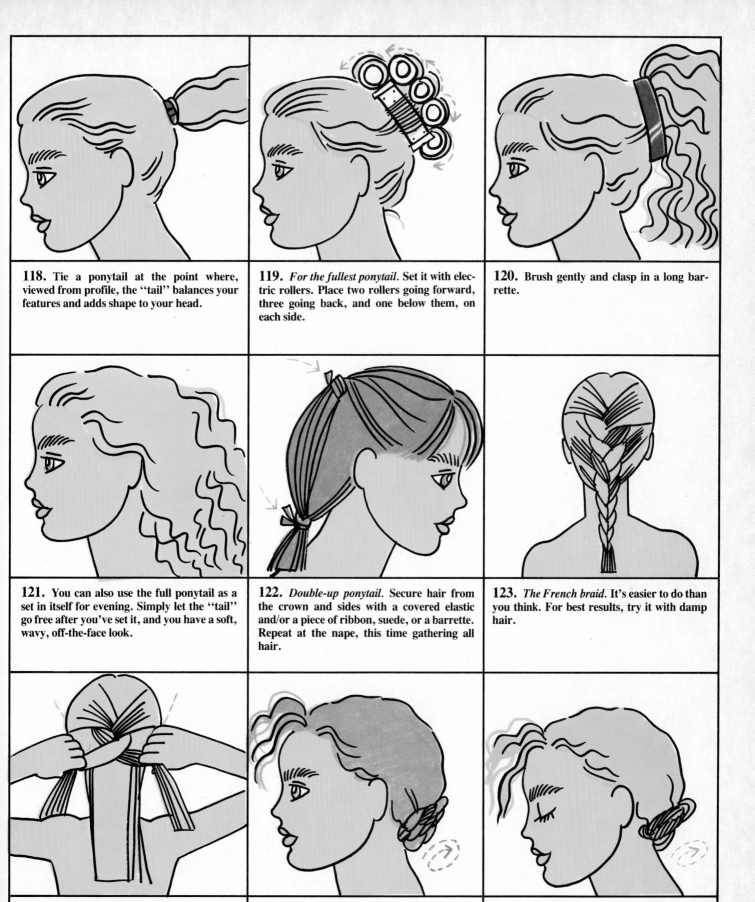

118. Tie a ponytail at the point where, viewed from profile, the "tail" balances your features and adds shape to your head.

119. *For the fullest ponytail.* Set it with electric rollers. Place two rollers going forward, three going back, and one below them, on each side.

120. Brush gently and clasp in a long barrette.

121. You can also use the full ponytail as a set in itself for evening. Simply let the "tail" go free after you've set it, and you have a soft, wavy, off-the-face look.

122. *Double-up ponytail.* Secure hair from the crown and sides with a covered elastic and/or a piece of ribbon, suede, or a barrette. Repeat at the nape, this time gathering all hair.

123. *The French braid.* It's easier to do than you think. For best results, try it with damp hair.

124. The method: divide your hair with a part across the top of your head, from ear to ear. Start braiding this top section. When you get down to ear level, braid in the remaining hair one section at a time.

125. *The braided twist.* Bring a few wisps of hair forward for softness, then bring the remaining hair back, softly braid, and gently twist/coil ends into a chignon at nape. Secure at nape with pins.

126. *The simple twist:* just twist the hair gently—don't braid it as in #125—and coil at the nape into a chignon. Secure with pins.

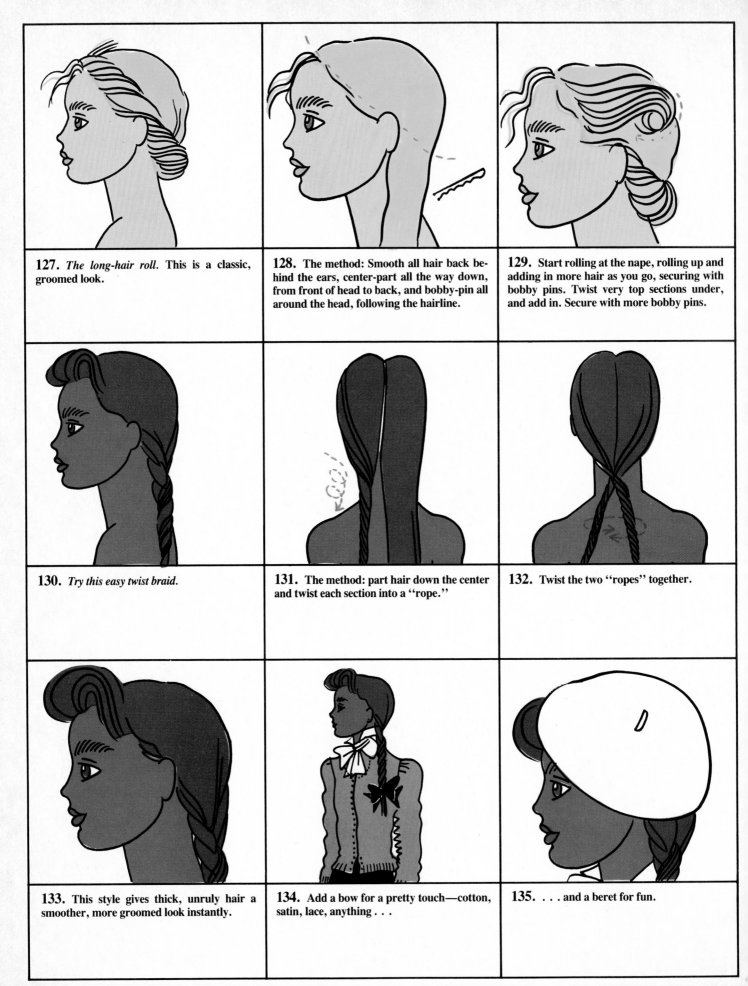

127. *The long-hair roll.* This is a classic, groomed look.

128. The method: Smooth all hair back behind the ears, center-part all the way down, from front of head to back, and bobby-pin all around the head, following the hairline.

129. Start rolling at the nape, rolling up and adding in more hair as you go, securing with bobby pins. Twist very top sections under, and add in. Secure with more bobby pins.

130. *Try this easy twist braid.*

131. The method: part hair down the center and twist each section into a "rope."

132. Twist the two "ropes" together.

133. This style gives thick, unruly hair a smoother, more groomed look instantly.

134. Add a bow for a pretty touch—cotton, satin, lace, anything . . .

135. . . . and a beret for fun.

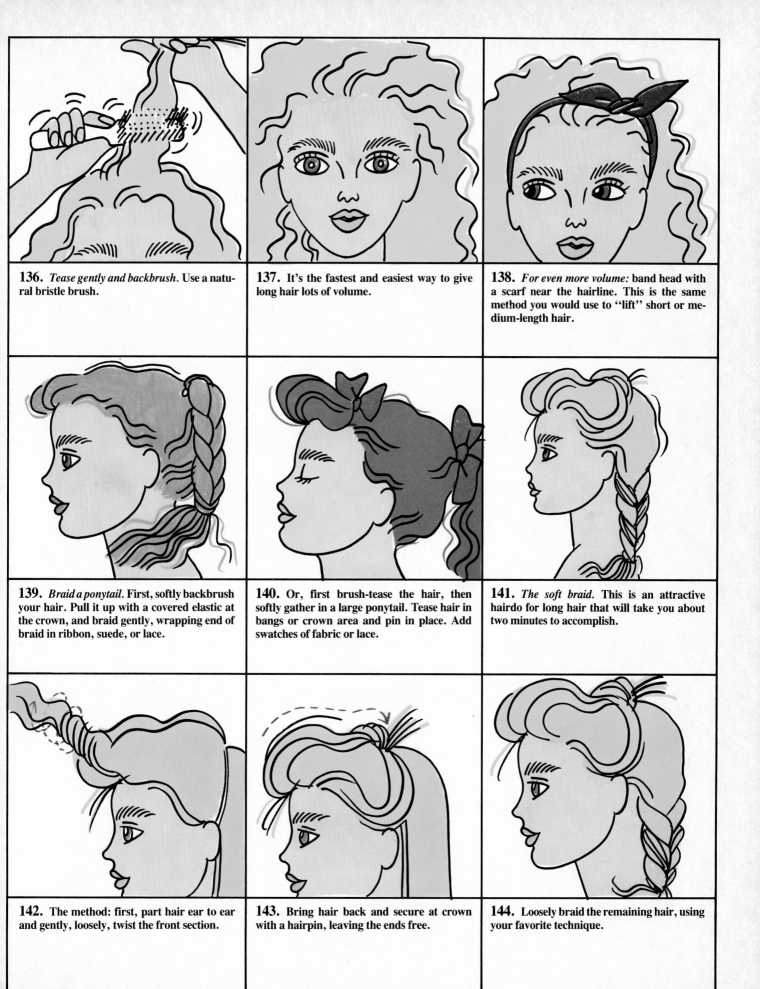

136. *Tease gently and backbrush.* Use a natural bristle brush.

137. It's the fastest and easiest way to give long hair lots of volume.

138. *For even more volume:* band head with a scarf near the hairline. This is the same method you would use to "lift" short or medium-length hair.

139. *Braid a ponytail.* First, softly backbrush your hair. Pull it up with a covered elastic at the crown, and braid gently, wrapping end of braid in ribbon, suede, or lace.

140. Or, first brush-tease the hair, then softly gather in a large ponytail. Tease hair in bangs or crown area and pin in place. Add swatches of fabric or lace.

141. *The soft braid.* This is an attractive hairdo for long hair that will take you about two minutes to accomplish.

142. The method: first, part hair ear to ear and gently, loosely, twist the front section.

143. Bring hair back and secure at crown with a hairpin, leaving the ends free.

144. Loosely braid the remaining hair, using your favorite technique.

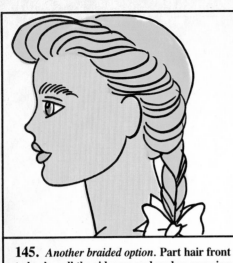

145. *Another braided option.* Part hair front to back, roll the sides up and under, securing with bobby pins where needed, and braid the remainder. Add a soft bow at the ends.

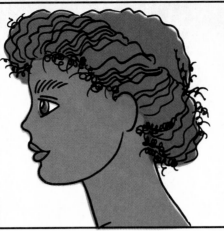

146. *Roll curly long hair.* You will get instant shape and polish.

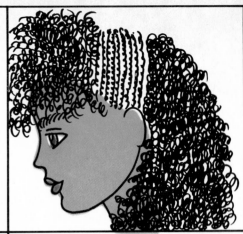

147. *Or, lift sides smoothly up.* Secure at top with pins and leave crown and remainder of hair free. Partial smoothness somewhere will give you a more controlled look.

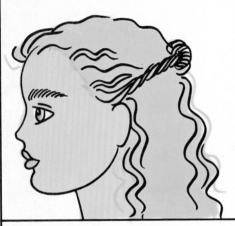

148. *An instant groomer.* This is a "young" look. It will also open up your face and emphasize your cheekbones.

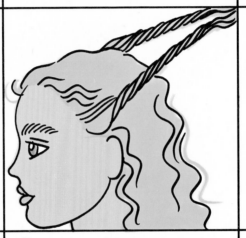

149. The method: twist side sections of hair back, coil together, and secure at the back with hairpins.

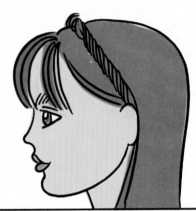

150. *Make a natural hairband.*

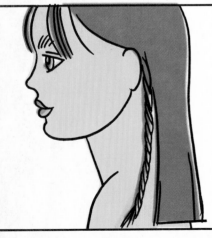

151. The method: take a section of hair on each side of your head, from right behind the ears, twist, lift to crown, and pin in a band.

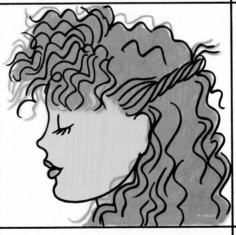

152. This technique works for long hair of every texture—straight, wavy, and curly.

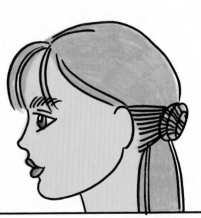

153. *The natural hairband modified.*

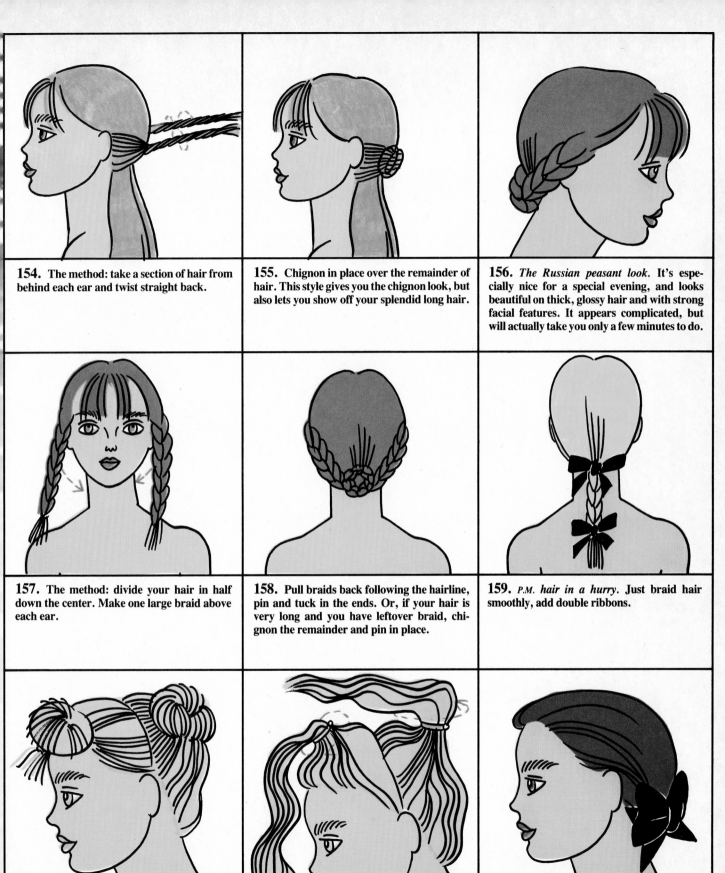

154. The method: take a section of hair from behind each ear and twist straight back.

155. Chignon in place over the remainder of hair. This style gives you the chignon look, but also lets you show off your splendid long hair.

156. *The Russian peasant look*. It's especially nice for a special evening, and looks beautiful on thick, glossy hair and with strong facial features. It appears complicated, but will actually take you only a few minutes to do.

157. The method: divide your hair in half down the center. Make one large braid above each ear.

158. Pull braids back following the hairline, pin and tuck in the ends. Or, if your hair is very long and you have leftover braid, chignon the remainder and pin in place.

159. *P.M. hair in a hurry*. Just braid hair smoothly, add double ribbons.

160. *An original style for evening*. When you find your hair collapsing . . .

161. . . . simply part hair ear to ear, loosely secure the front and back sections with a covered elastic, about 2″ above the scalp, then twist and coil ends in two chignons, securing with pins.

162. *Easy elegance*. Smooth all hair back, add a touch of pure lanolin for sheen, and chignon or knot at nape. Add a huge black velvet bow.

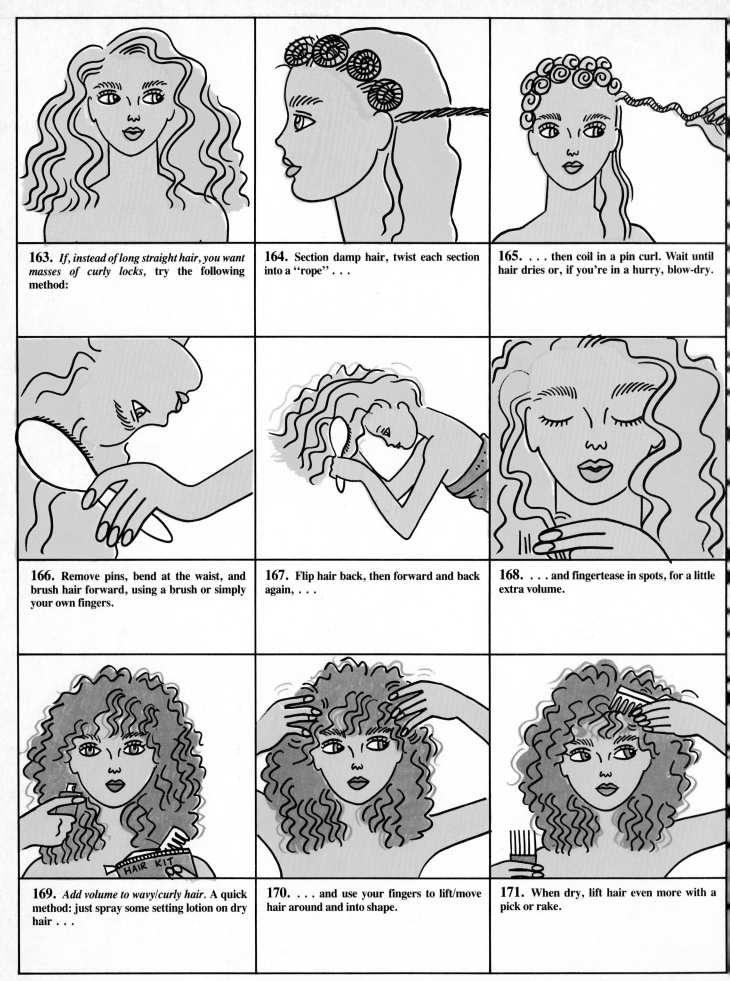

163. *If, instead of long straight hair, you want masses of curly locks,* try the following method:

164. Section damp hair, twist each section into a "rope" . . .

165. . . . then coil in a pin curl. Wait until hair dries or, if you're in a hurry, blow-dry.

166. Remove pins, bend at the waist, and brush hair forward, using a brush or simply your own fingers.

167. Flip hair back, then forward and back again, . . .

168. . . . and fingertease in spots, for a little extra volume.

169. *Add volume to wavy/curly hair.* A quick method: just spray some setting lotion on dry hair . . .

170. . . . and use your fingers to lift/move hair around and into shape.

171. When dry, lift hair even more with a pick or rake.

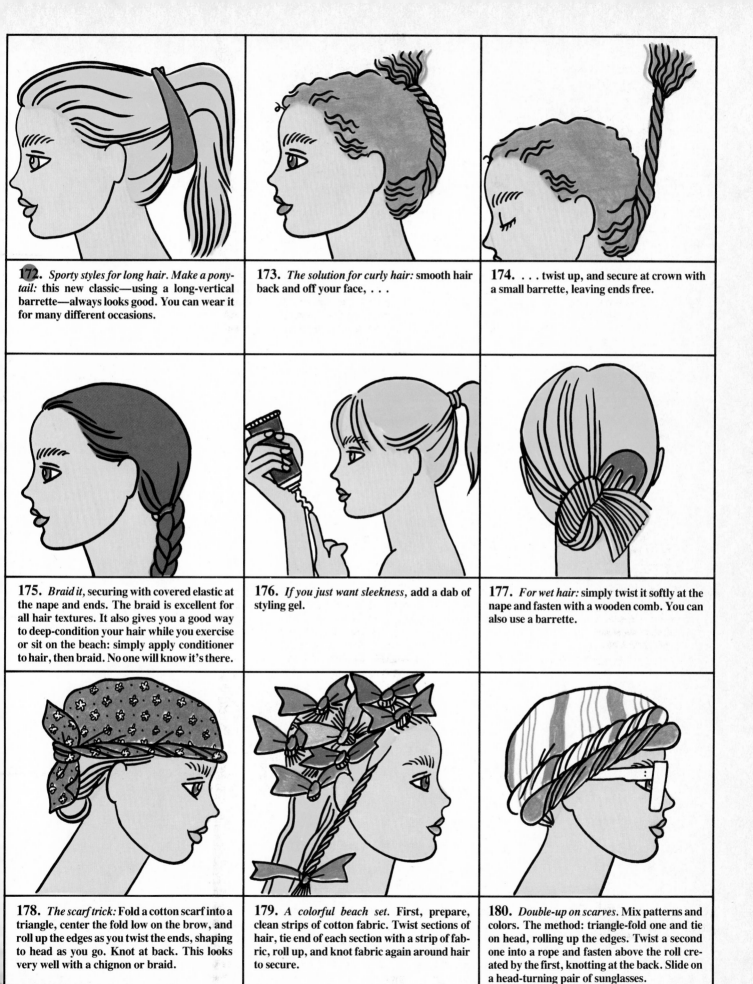

172. *Sporty styles for long hair.* Make a pony-tail: this new classic—using a long-vertical barrette—always looks good. You can wear it for many different occasions.

173. *The solution for curly hair:* smooth hair back and off your face, . . .

174. . . . twist up, and secure at crown with a small barrette, leaving ends free.

175. *Braid it,* securing with covered elastic at the nape and ends. The braid is excellent for all hair textures. It also gives you a good way to deep-condition your hair while you exercise or sit on the beach: simply apply conditioner to hair, then braid. No one will know it's there.

176. *If you just want sleekness,* add a dab of styling gel.

177. *For wet hair:* simply twist it softly at the nape and fasten with a wooden comb. You can also use a barrette.

178. *The scarf trick:* Fold a cotton scarf into a triangle, center the fold low on the brow, and roll up the edges as you twist the ends, shaping to head as you go. Knot at back. This looks very well with a chignon or braid.

179. *A colorful beach set.* First, prepare, clean strips of cotton fabric. Twist sections of hair, tie end of each section with a strip of fabric, roll up, and knot fabric again around hair to secure.

180. *Double-up on scarves.* Mix patterns and colors. The method: triangle-fold one and tie on head, rolling up the edges. Twist a second one into a rope and fasten above the roll created by the first, knotting at the back. Slide on a head-turning pair of sunglasses.

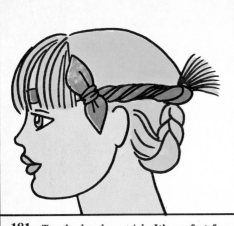

181. *Try the bandana trick.* It's perfect for medium or long hair with bangs. Braid hair in the back, twist a dampened cotton bandana, and circle your head with it, going under the bangs and lifting up the braid. Knot on the side.

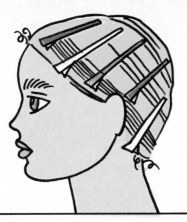

182. *Use your head as one giant roller.* For sleek hair, brush it while completely wet in one direction, all around your head, clipping it in place as you go. Dry, then remove clips.

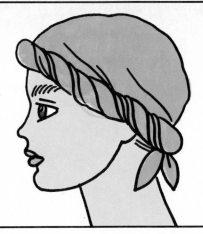

183. *The peasant look.* Place a soft, thin piece of fabric or a scarf on your head and roll the edges, bringing fabric down over the ears. Knot at back.

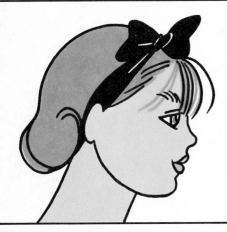

184. *The easy pageboy.* All you need is a soft ribbon. Chiffon would be fine.

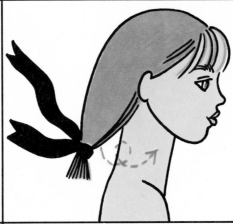

185. The method: knot ribbon at ends of the hair.

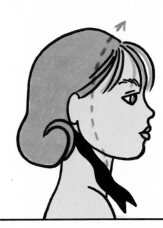

186. Roll hair under, bringing the ends of the ribbon up on both sides, and tie them at the crown.

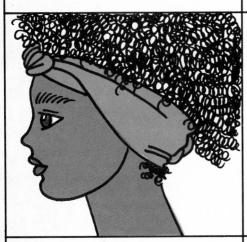

187. *Tie it up with a piece of stretchy fabric.* It will take hair off your face and create a wonderful, unusual look. It also absorbs perspiration.

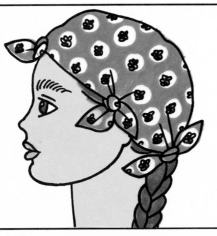

188. *For playtime:* knot a scarf at the corners, place on your head, and knot again to pull tighter and adjust. You should end up with three or four knots.

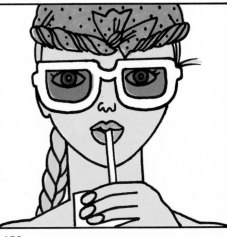

189. *If you wear scarves with glasses:* make sure you place the scarf higher on your forehead, and leave the ears exposed.

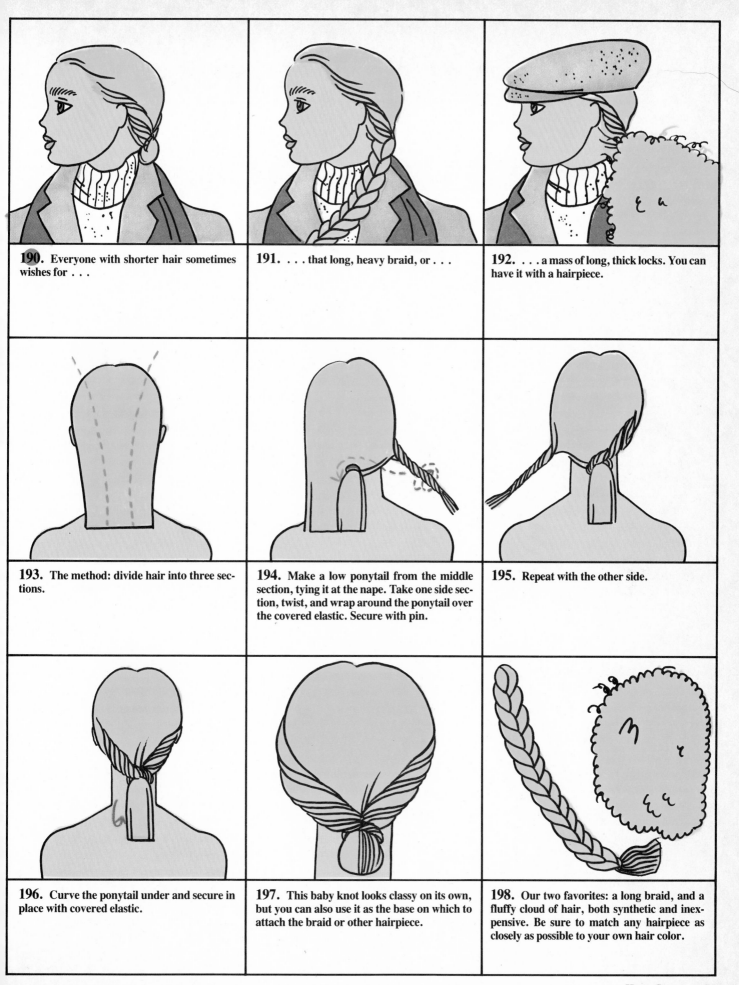

190. Everyone with shorter hair sometimes wishes for . . .

191. . . . that long, heavy braid, or . . .

192. . . . a mass of long, thick locks. You can have it with a hairpiece.

193. The method: divide hair into three sections.

194. Make a low ponytail from the middle section, tying it at the nape. Take one side section, twist, and wrap around the ponytail over the covered elastic. Secure with pin.

195. Repeat with the other side.

196. Curve the ponytail under and secure in place with covered elastic.

197. This baby knot looks classy on its own, but you can also use it as the base on which to attach the braid or other hairpiece.

198. Our two favorites: a long braid, and a fluffy cloud of hair, both synthetic and inexpensive. Be sure to match any hairpiece as closely as possible to your own hair color.

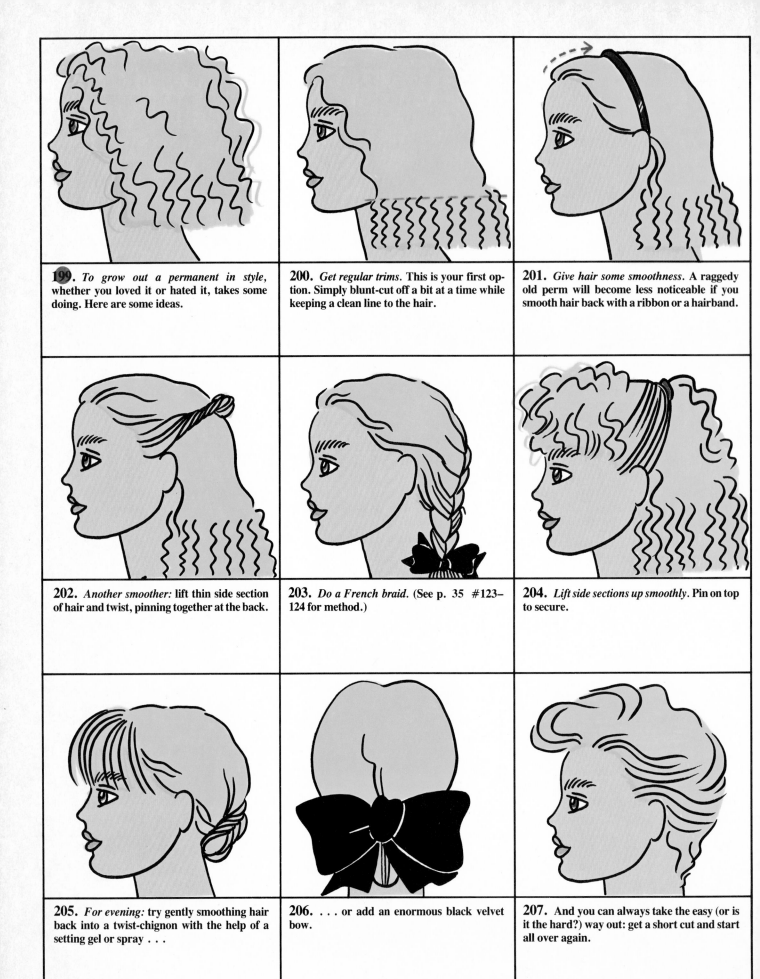

199. *To grow out a permanent in style,* whether you loved it or hated it, takes some doing. Here are some ideas.

200. *Get regular trims.* This is your first option. Simply blunt-cut off a bit at a time while keeping a clean line to the hair.

201. *Give hair some smoothness.* A raggedy old perm will become less noticeable if you smooth hair back with a ribbon or a hairband.

202. *Another smoother:* lift thin side section of hair and twist, pinning together at the back.

203. *Do a French braid.* (See p. 35 #123–124 for method.)

204. *Lift side sections up smoothly.* Pin on top to secure.

205. *For evening:* try gently smoothing hair back into a twist-chignon with the help of a setting gel or spray . . .

206. . . . or add an enormous black velvet bow.

207. And you can always take the easy (or is it the hard?) way out: get a short cut and start all over again.

5
BODY CARE

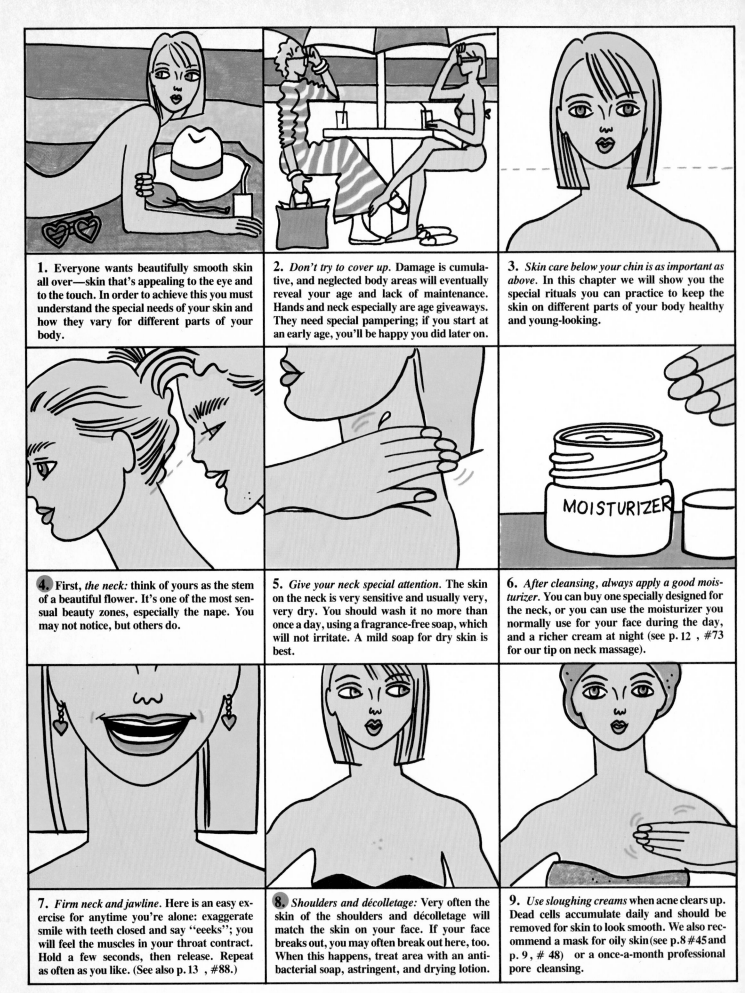

1. **Everyone wants beautifully smooth skin all over—skin that's appealing to the eye and to the touch.** In order to achieve this you must understand the special needs of your skin and how they vary for different parts of your body.

2. *Don't try to cover up.* Damage is cumulative, and neglected body areas will eventually reveal your age and lack of maintenance. Hands and neck especially are age giveaways. They need special pampering; if you start at an early age, you'll be happy you did later on.

3. *Skin care below your chin is as important as above.* In this chapter we will show you the special rituals you can practice to keep the skin on different parts of your body healthy and young-looking.

4. First, *the neck:* think of yours as the stem of a beautiful flower. It's one of the most sensual beauty zones, especially the nape. You may not notice, but others do.

5. *Give your neck special attention.* The skin on the neck is very sensitive and usually very, very dry. You should wash it no more than once a day, using a fragrance-free soap, which will not irritate. A mild soap for dry skin is best.

6. *After cleansing, always apply a good moisturizer.* You can buy one specially designed for the neck, or you can use the moisturizer you normally use for your face during the day, and a richer cream at night (see p. 12 , #73 for our tip on neck massage).

7. *Firm neck and jawline.* Here is an easy exercise for anytime you're alone: exaggerate smile with teeth closed and say "eeeks"; you will feel the muscles in your throat contract. Hold a few seconds, then release. Repeat as often as you like. (See also p. 13 , #88.)

8. *Shoulders and décolletage:* Very often the skin of the shoulders and décolletage will match the skin on your face. If your face breaks out, you may often break out here, too. When this happens, treat area with an antibacterial soap, astringent, and drying lotion.

9. *Use sloughing creams* when acne clears up. Dead cells accumulate daily and should be removed for skin to look smooth. We also recommend a mask for oily skin (see p. 8 #45 and p. 9 , # 48) or a once-a-month professional pore cleansing.

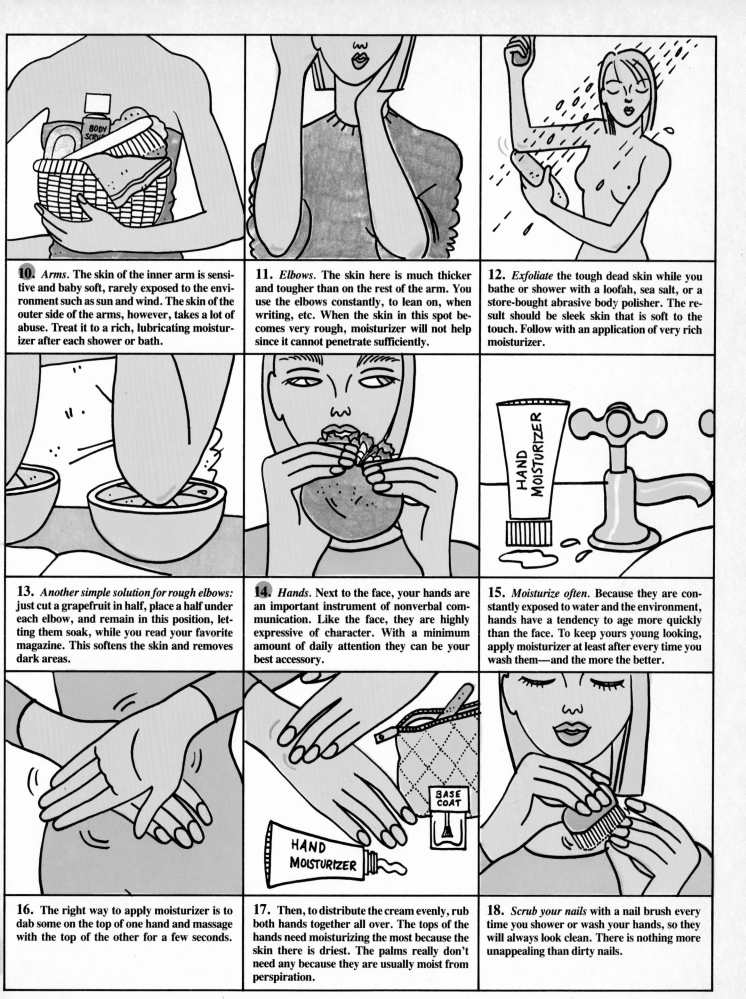

10. *Arms.* The skin of the inner arm is sensitive and baby soft, rarely exposed to the environment such as sun and wind. The skin of the outer side of the arms, however, takes a lot of abuse. Treat it to a rich, lubricating moisturizer after each shower or bath.

11. *Elbows.* The skin here is much thicker and tougher than on the rest of the arm. You use the elbows constantly, to lean on, when writing, etc. When the skin in this spot becomes very rough, moisturizer will not help since it cannot penetrate sufficiently.

12. *Exfoliate* the tough dead skin while you bathe or shower with a loofah, sea salt, or a store-bought abrasive body polisher. The result should be sleek skin that is soft to the touch. Follow with an application of very rich moisturizer.

13. *Another simple solution for rough elbows:* just cut a grapefruit in half, place a half under each elbow, and remain in this position, letting them soak, while you read your favorite magazine. This softens the skin and removes dark areas.

14. *Hands.* Next to the face, your hands are an important instrument of nonverbal communication. Like the face, they are highly expressive of character. With a minimum amount of daily attention they can be your best accessory.

15. *Moisturize often.* Because they are constantly exposed to water and the environment, hands have a tendency to age more quickly than the face. To keep yours young looking, apply moisturizer at least after every time you wash them—and the more the better.

16. The right way to apply moisturizer is to dab some on the top of one hand and massage with the top of the other for a few seconds.

17. Then, to distribute the cream evenly, rub both hands together all over. The tops of the hands need moisturizing the most because the skin there is driest. The palms really don't need any because they are usually moist from perspiration.

18. *Scrub your nails* with a nail brush every time you shower or wash your hands, so they will always look clean. There is nothing more unappealing than dirty nails.

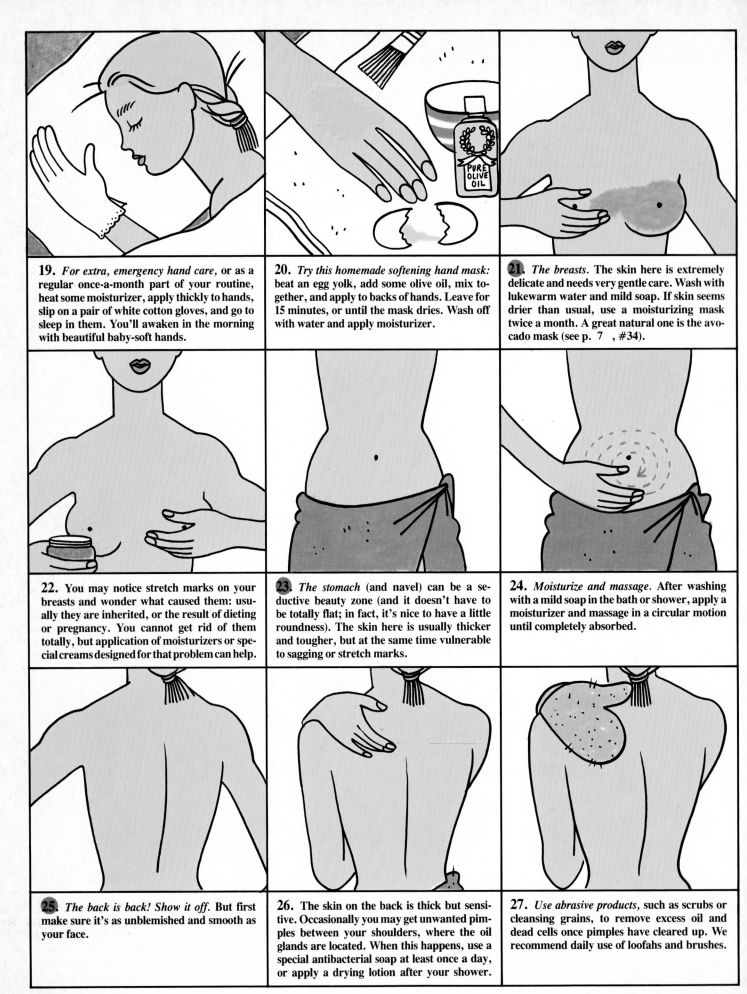

19. *For extra, emergency hand care,* or as a regular once-a-month part of your routine, heat some moisturizer, apply thickly to hands, slip on a pair of white cotton gloves, and go to sleep in them. You'll awaken in the morning with beautiful baby-soft hands.

20. *Try this homemade softening hand mask:* beat an egg yolk, add some olive oil, mix together, and apply to backs of hands. Leave for 15 minutes, or until the mask dries. Wash off with water and apply moisturizer.

21. *The breasts.* The skin here is extremely delicate and needs very gentle care. Wash with lukewarm water and mild soap. If skin seems drier than usual, use a moisturizing mask twice a month. A great natural one is the avocado mask (see p. 7 , #34).

22. You may notice stretch marks on your breasts and wonder what caused them: usually they are inherited, or the result of dieting or pregnancy. You cannot get rid of them totally, but application of moisturizers or special creams designed for that problem can help.

23. *The stomach* (and navel) can be a seductive beauty zone (and it doesn't have to be totally flat; in fact, it's nice to have a little roundness). The skin here is usually thicker and tougher, but at the same time vulnerable to sagging or stretch marks.

24. *Moisturize and massage.* After washing with a mild soap in the bath or shower, apply a moisturizer and massage in a circular motion until completely absorbed.

25. *The back is back! Show it off.* But first make sure it's as unblemished and smooth as your face.

26. The skin on the back is thick but sensitive. Occasionally you may get unwanted pimples between your shoulders, where the oil glands are located. When this happens, use a special antibacterial soap at least once a day, or apply a drying lotion after your shower.

27. *Use abrasive products,* such as scrubs or cleansing grains, to remove excess oil and dead cells once pimples have cleared up. We recommend daily use of loofahs and brushes.

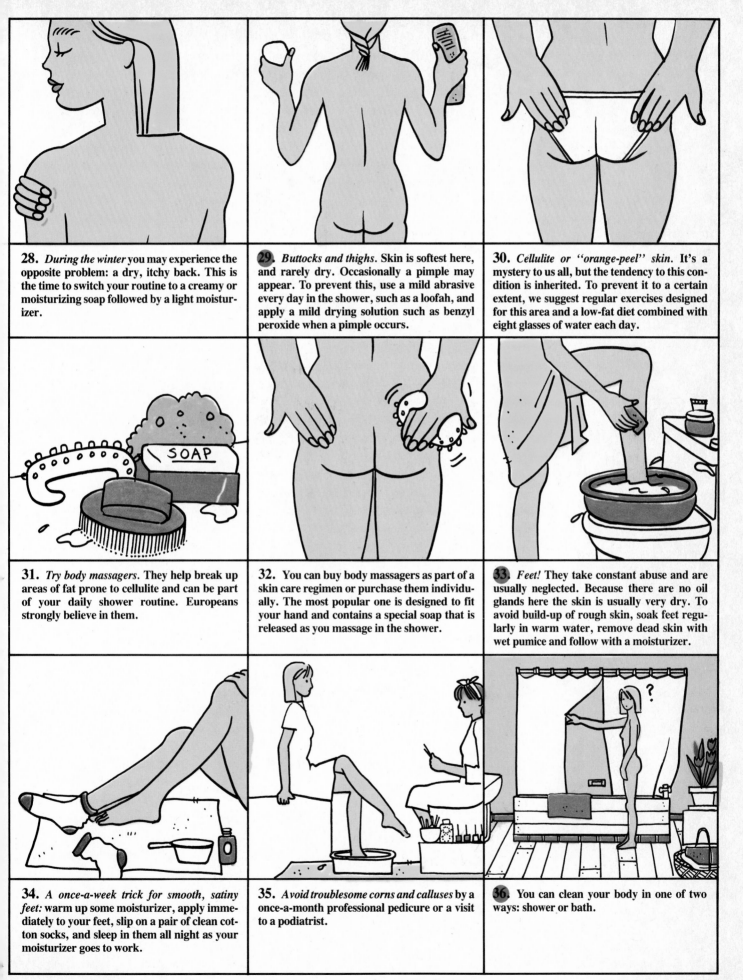

28. *During the winter* you may experience the opposite problem: a dry, itchy back. This is the time to switch your routine to a creamy or moisturizing soap followed by a light moisturizer.

29. *Buttocks and thighs.* Skin is softest here, and rarely dry. Occasionally a pimple may appear. To prevent this, use a mild abrasive every day in the shower, such as a loofah, and apply a mild drying solution such as benzyl peroxide when a pimple occurs.

30. *Cellulite or "orange-peel" skin.* It's a mystery to us all, but the tendency to this condition is inherited. To prevent it to a certain extent, we suggest regular exercises designed for this area and a low-fat diet combined with eight glasses of water each day.

31. *Try body massagers.* They help break up areas of fat prone to cellulite and can be part of your daily shower routine. Europeans strongly believe in them.

32. You can buy body massagers as part of a skin care regimen or purchase them individually. The most popular one is designed to fit your hand and contains a special soap that is released as you massage in the shower.

33. *Feet!* They take constant abuse and are usually neglected. Because there are no oil glands here the skin is usually very dry. To avoid build-up of rough skin, soak feet regularly in warm water, remove dead skin with wet pumice and follow with a moisturizer.

34. *A once-a-week trick for smooth, satiny feet:* warm up some moisturizer, apply immediately to your feet, slip on a pair of clean cotton socks, and sleep in them all night as your moisturizer goes to work.

35. *Avoid troublesome corns and calluses* by a once-a-month professional pedicure or a visit to a podiatrist.

36. You can clean your body in one of two ways: shower or bath.

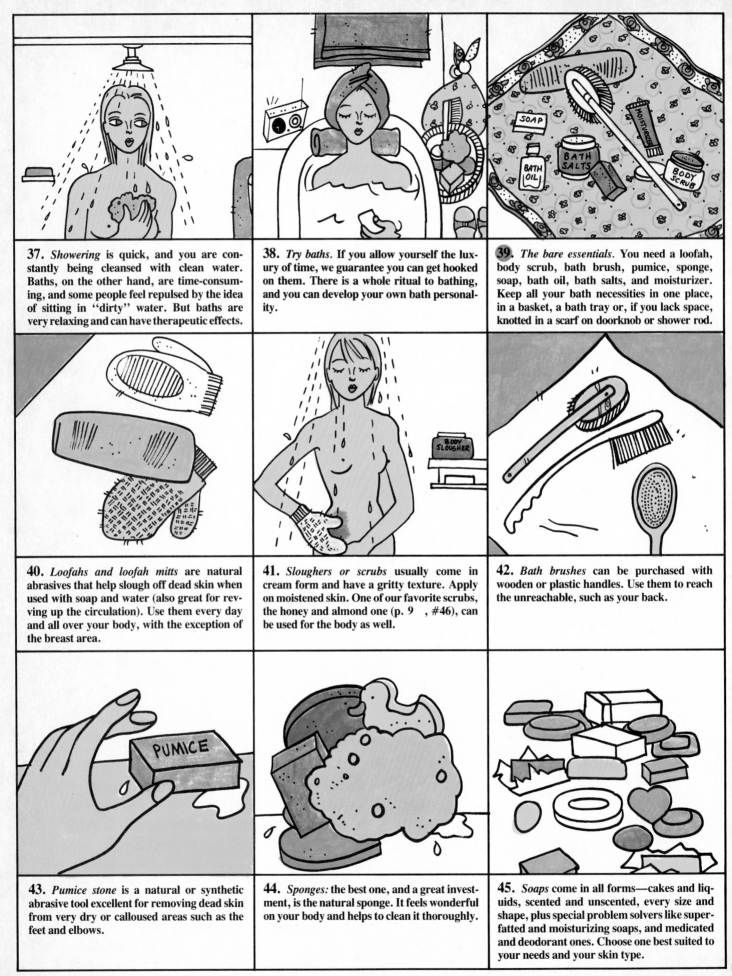

37. *Showering* is quick, and you are constantly being cleansed with clean water. Baths, on the other hand, are time-consuming, and some people feel repulsed by the idea of sitting in "dirty" water. But baths are very relaxing and can have therapeutic effects.

38. *Try baths.* If you allow yourself the luxury of time, we guarantee you can get hooked on them. There is a whole ritual to bathing, and you can develop your own bath personality.

39. *The bare essentials.* You need a loofah, body scrub, bath brush, pumice, sponge, soap, bath oil, bath salts, and moisturizer. Keep all your bath necessities in one place, in a basket, a bath tray or, if you lack space, knotted in a scarf on doorknob or shower rod.

40. *Loofahs and loofah mitts* are natural abrasives that help slough off dead skin when used with soap and water (also great for revving up the circulation). Use them every day and all over your body, with the exception of the breast area.

41. *Sloughers or scrubs* usually come in cream form and have a gritty texture. Apply on moistened skin. One of our favorite scrubs, the honey and almond one (p. 9 , #46), can be used for the body as well.

42. *Bath brushes* can be purchased with wooden or plastic handles. Use them to reach the unreachable, such as your back.

43. *Pumice stone* is a natural or synthetic abrasive tool excellent for removing dead skin from very dry or calloused areas such as the feet and elbows.

44. *Sponges:* the best one, and a great investment, is the natural sponge. It feels wonderful on your body and helps to clean it thoroughly.

45. *Soaps* come in all forms—cakes and liquids, scented and unscented, every size and shape, plus special problem solvers like superfatted and moisturizing soaps, and medicated and deodorant ones. Choose one best suited to your needs and your skin type.

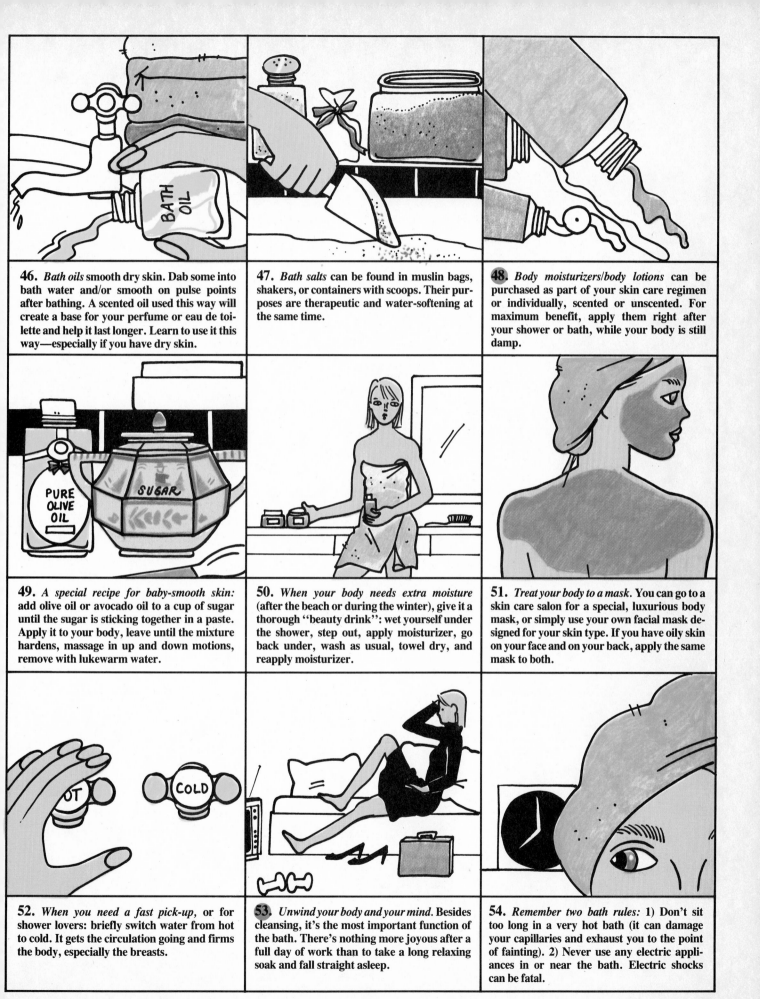

46. *Bath oils* smooth dry skin. Dab some into bath water and/or smooth on pulse points after bathing. A scented oil used this way will create a base for your perfume or eau de toilette and help it last longer. Learn to use it this way—especially if you have dry skin.

47. *Bath salts* can be found in muslin bags, shakers, or containers with scoops. Their purposes are therapeutic and water-softening at the same time.

48. *Body moisturizers/body lotions* can be purchased as part of your skin care regimen or individually, scented or unscented. For maximum benefit, apply them right after your shower or bath, while your body is still damp.

49. *A special recipe for baby-smooth skin:* add olive oil or avocado oil to a cup of sugar until the sugar is sticking together in a paste. Apply it to your body, leave until the mixture hardens, massage in up and down motions, remove with lukewarm water.

50. *When your body needs extra moisture* (after the beach or during the winter), give it a thorough "beauty drink": wet yourself under the shower, step out, apply moisturizer, go back under, wash as usual, towel dry, and reapply moisturizer.

51. *Treat your body to a mask.* You can go to a skin care salon for a special, luxurious body mask, or simply use your own facial mask designed for your skin type. If you have oily skin on your face and on your back, apply the same mask to both.

52. *When you need a fast pick-up,* or for shower lovers: briefly switch water from hot to cold. It gets the circulation going and firms the body, especially the breasts.

53. *Unwind your body and your mind.* Besides cleansing, it's the most important function of the bath. There's nothing more joyous after a full day of work than to take a long relaxing soak and fall straight asleep.

54. *Remember two bath rules:* 1) Don't sit too long in a very hot bath (it can damage your capillaries and exhaust you to the point of fainting). 2) Never use any electric appliances in or near the bath. Electric shocks can be fatal.

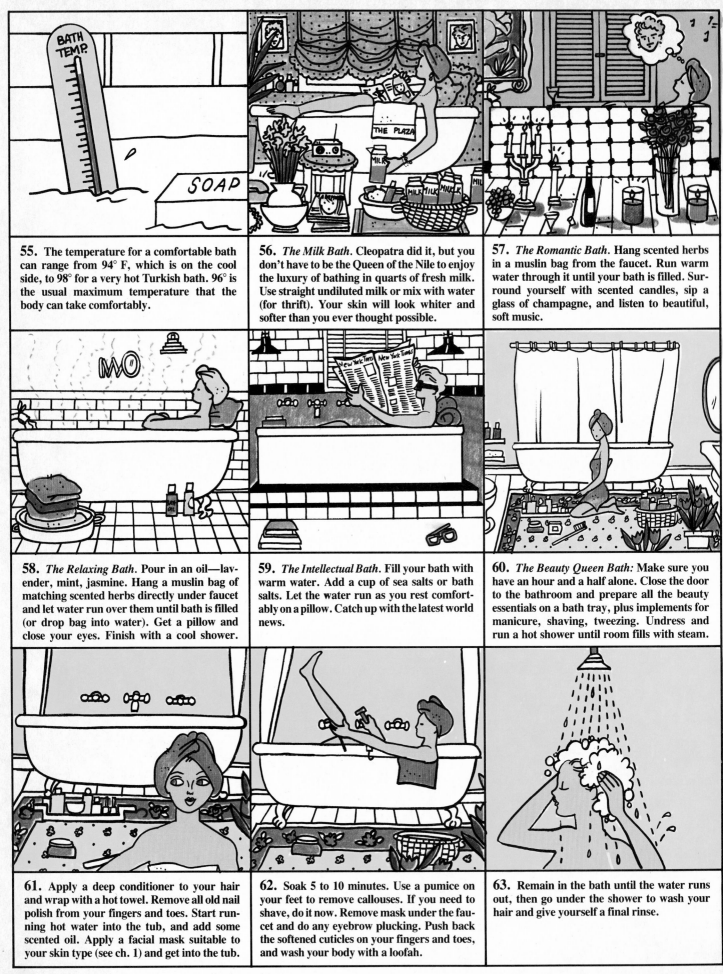

55. The temperature for a comfortable bath can range from 94° F, which is on the cool side, to 98° for a very hot Turkish bath. 96° is the usual maximum temperature that the body can take comfortably.

56. *The Milk Bath.* Cleopatra did it, but you don't have to be the Queen of the Nile to enjoy the luxury of bathing in quarts of fresh milk. Use straight undiluted milk or mix with water (for thrift). Your skin will look whiter and softer than you ever thought possible.

57. *The Romantic Bath.* Hang scented herbs in a muslin bag from the faucet. Run warm water through it until your bath is filled. Surround yourself with scented candles, sip a glass of champagne, and listen to beautiful, soft music.

58. *The Relaxing Bath.* Pour in an oil—lavender, mint, jasmine. Hang a muslin bag of matching scented herbs directly under faucet and let water run over them until bath is filled (or drop bag into water). Get a pillow and close your eyes. Finish with a cool shower.

59. *The Intellectual Bath.* Fill your bath with warm water. Add a cup of sea salts or bath salts. Let the water run as you rest comfortably on a pillow. Catch up with the latest world news.

60. *The Beauty Queen Bath:* Make sure you have an hour and a half alone. Close the door to the bathroom and prepare all the beauty essentials on a bath tray, plus implements for manicure, shaving, tweezing. Undress and run a hot shower until room fills with steam.

61. Apply a deep conditioner to your hair and wrap with a hot towel. Remove all old nail polish from your fingers and toes. Start running hot water into the tub, and add some scented oil. Apply a facial mask suitable to your skin type (see ch. 1) and get into the tub.

62. Soak 5 to 10 minutes. Use a pumice on your feet to remove callouses. If you need to shave, do it now. Remove mask under the faucet and do any eyebrow plucking. Push back the softened cuticles on your fingers and toes, and wash your body with a loofah.

63. Remain in the bath until the water runs out, then go under the shower to wash your hair and give yourself a final rinse.

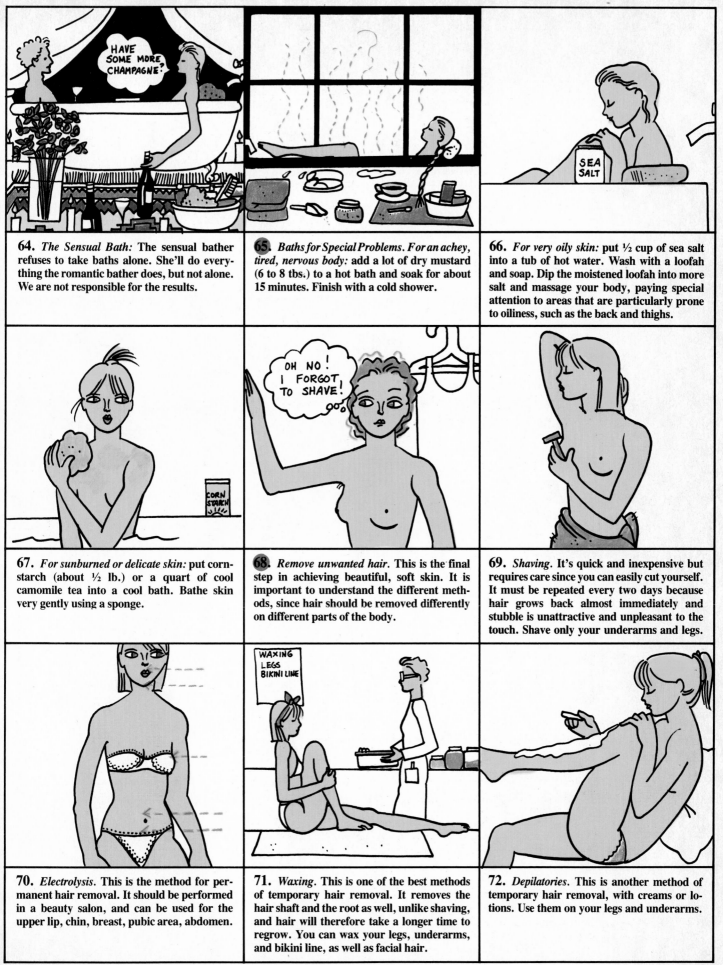

64. *The Sensual Bath:* The sensual bather refuses to take baths alone. She'll do everything the romantic bather does, but not alone. We are not responsible for the results.

65. *Baths for Special Problems. For an achey, tired, nervous body:* add a lot of dry mustard (6 to 8 tbs.) to a hot bath and soak for about 15 minutes. Finish with a cold shower.

66. *For very oily skin:* put ½ cup of sea salt into a tub of hot water. Wash with a loofah and soap. Dip the moistened loofah into more salt and massage your body, paying special attention to areas that are particularly prone to oiliness, such as the back and thighs.

67. *For sunburned or delicate skin:* put cornstarch (about ½ lb.) or a quart of cool camomile tea into a cool bath. Bathe skin very gently using a sponge.

68. *Remove unwanted hair.* This is the final step in achieving beautiful, soft skin. It is important to understand the different methods, since hair should be removed differently on different parts of the body.

69. *Shaving.* It's quick and inexpensive but requires care since you can easily cut yourself. It must be repeated every two days because hair grows back almost immediately and stubble is unattractive and unpleasant to the touch. Shave only your underarms and legs.

70. *Electrolysis.* This is the method for permanent hair removal. It should be performed in a beauty salon, and can be used for the upper lip, chin, breast, pubic area, abdomen.

71. *Waxing.* This is one of the best methods of temporary hair removal. It removes the hair shaft and the root as well, unlike shaving, and hair will therefore take a longer time to regrow. You can wax your legs, underarms, and bikini line, as well as facial hair.

72. *Depilatories.* This is another method of temporary hair removal, with creams or lotions. Use them on your legs and underarms.

Afterword

Beauty, like fashion, rests on certain fundamental principles—a number of rules and how-to's that remain the same regardless of the particular styles that prevail at a given moment. It is these rules—the basics of a sensible, effective beauty regimen—that we have presented in this book. Once you know them, feel free to experiment; keep them in mind and you will always look your best.

Index

About the authors:

FELICIA MILEWICZ joined *Mademoiselle Magazine* in 1971. She has worked as Assistant to the Sportswear Editor and the Shoes Editor, as the Models Editor, and since 1977 she has been the magazine's Beauty and Health Editor. She is responsible for approximately twenty pages of each month's issue, developing articles on beauty, diet, health and exercise, and works on a regular basis with the country's foremost skin, hair, make-up and exercise experts, as well as with the top fashion models and photographers. She lives in New York City with her husband and son.

LOIS JOY JOHNSON joined *Mademoiselle* in 1979 as Assistant Beauty Editor after a ten-year career as a free-lance fashion and beauty illustrator. In September 1982 she was appointed Beauty and Fashion Editor of *Ladies' Home Journal*. She is responsible for developing and producing all stories related to beauty, fashion, health and fitness each month, and works daily with the top specialists in these fields. She lives with her daughter in New York.